Frontiers of Radiation Therapy and Oncology

Vol. 16

Editor
Jerome M. Vaeth, San Francisco, Calif.

Associate Editors
Jerold P. Green, *Alan F. Schröder*, *Simeon T. Cantril* and
Mary Louise Meurk

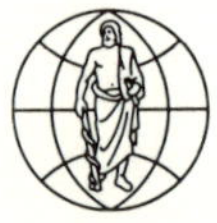

S. Karger · Basel · München · Paris · London · New York · Sydney

16th Annual San Francisco Cancer Symposium, San Francisco, Calif.
March 13–14, 1981

Childhood Cancer: Triumph over Tragedy

Editor
Jerome M. Vaeth, San Francisco, Calif.

36 figures and 32 tables, 1982

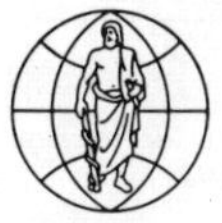

S. Karger · Basel · München · Paris · London · New York · Sydney

Frontiers of Radiation Therapy and Oncology

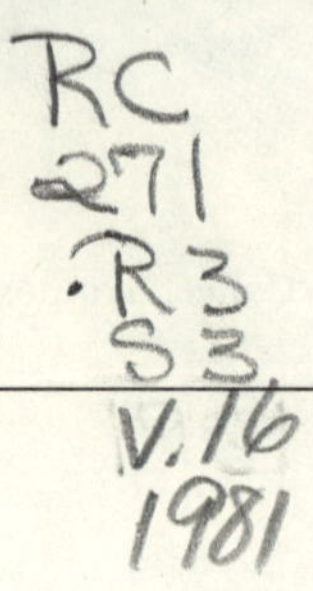

Vol. 14: Body Image, Self-Esteem, and Sexuality in Cancer Patients. 14th Annual San Francisco Cancer Symposium, San Francisco, Calif., 1979. J.M. Vaeth, R.C. Blomberg and L. Adler, San Francisco, Calif. (eds.)
X + 134 p., 16 fig., 6 tab., 1980. ISBN 3-8055-0036-X
Vol. 15: Pharmaceutical Aspects of Cancer Care. 15th Annual San Francisco Cancer Symposium, San Francisco, Calif., 1980. J.M. Vaeth, San Francisco, Calif. (ed.)
VIII + 184 p., 20 fig., 61 tab., 1981. ISBN 3-8055-1512-X

National Library of Medicine, Cataloging in Publication
San Francisco Cancer Symposium (16th; 1981)
Childhood Cancer, triumph over tragedy: 16th annual San Francisco Cancer Symposium, San Francisco, Calif., March 13-14, 1981
Editor, Jerome M. Vaeth. – Basel, New York, Karger, 1982.
(Frontiers of radiation therapy and oncology; v. 16)
1. Neoplasms – in infancy and childhood – congresses I. Vaeth, Jerome M., 1925 – II. Title III. Series
W3 FR 935 v.16/QZ 200 S195 1981c
ISBN 3-8055-3020-X

Drug Dosage

The author and publisher have exerted every effort to ensure that drug selection and dosage set forth in this text are in accord with current recommendations and practice at the time of publication. However, in view of ongoing research, changes in government regulations, and the constant flow of information relating to drug therapy and drug reactions, the reader is urged to check the package insert for each drug for any change in indications and dosage and for added warnings and precautions. This is particularly important when the recommended agent is a new and/or infrequently employed drug.

Contents

Carter, S.K. (Palo Alto, Calif.): Introduction 1

Austin, D.F.; Nelson V.E.; Johnson, L.F. (Oakland, Calif.): Epidemiologic Characteristics of Childhood Cancer 9

Evans, A.E. (Philadelphia, Pa.): Leukemia: Historical Development of Cancer Therapy. The First Battle is Won 18

D'Angio, G.; Evans, A.; Breslow, N.; Baum, E.; Beckwith, J.B.; deLorimier, A.; Fernbach, D.; Hrabovsky, E.; Jones, B.; Kelalis, P.; Othersen, H.B. Jr.; Tefft, M.; Thomas, P. (Philadelphia, Pa. / Seattle, Wash. / Chicago, Ill. / San Francisco, Calif. / Houston, Tex. / Morgantown, W.Va. / Rochester, Minn. / Charleston, S.C. / Providence, R.I. / St. Louis, Mo.): Management of Children with Wilms' Tumor: Defining the Risk-Benefit Ratio 30

Discussion 40

Glaubiger D.L.; von Hoff, D.D.; Holcenberg, J.S.; Kamen, B.; Pratt, C.; Ungerleider, R.S. (Bethesda, Md. / San Antonio, Tex. / Milwaukee, Wisc.): The Relative Tolerance of Children and Adults to Anticancer Drugs 42

Bleyer, W.A. (Seattle, Wash.): Delayed Toxicities of Chemotherapy on Childhood Tissues. 1981 Update 50

Meyskens, F.L. Jr. (Tucson, Ariz.): Individualized Patient Chemotherapy: Use of a Human Tumor Colony Formation Technique 55

Rubin, P.; Van Houtte, P.; Constine, L. (Rochester, N.Y.): Radiation Sensitivity and Organ Tolerances in Pediatric Oncology: A New Hypothesis 62

Discussion 83

Johnson, F.L. (Seattle, Wash.): Bone Marrow Transplants 86

Bloom, H.J.G. (London): Brain Gliomas in Children: Treatment Policy and Prognosis 90

Jaffe, N. (Houston, Tex.): Malignant Bone Tumors in Children. A Decade of Progress 105

Hays, D.M. (Los Angeles, Calif.): Soft Tissue Sarcomas in Childhood 114

Donaldson, S.S. (Stanford, Calif.): Hodgkin's Disease. Treatment with Low Dose Radiation and Chemotherapy 122

Contents   VI

*Jenkin, R.D.T.; Anderson, J.R.; Chilcote, R.R.; Coccia, P.; Exelby, P.; Kersey, J.;
    Kushner, J.; Meadows, A.; Siegel, S.; Wilson, J.; Leiken, S.; Hammond, D.*
    (Los Angeles, Calif.): Paediatric Non-Hodgkin's Lymphomas: The Chil-
    drens' Cancer Study Group Experience. An Interim Report 134
Ablin, A.R. (San Francisco, Calif.): Malignant Germ Cell Tumors in Children ... 141
Kushner, J.H. (San Francisco, Calif.): Histiocytosis X 150
Discussion.. 153
Bartholome, W.G. (Houston, Tex.): The Ethical Rights of the Child Patient 156
Spinetta, J.J. (San Diego, Calif.): Impact of Cancer on the Family.............. 167
Eys, J. van (Houston, Tex.): Nutrition of Children with Cancer 177
Brown, H.G. (Los Angeles, Calif.): Unorthodox Methods of Treatment for
    Cancer 184
Discussion.. 190

Forword

The 16th Annual San Francisco Cancer Symposium was entitled 'Childhood Cancer: Triumph over Tragedy'. In years past, but with few exceptions, children with cancer died, and the parents were emotionally maimed. Today, through the joint efforts of the oncological specialists – surgical, radiation and medical – children formerly doomed are alive and free of cancer. The foremost oncologic specialists in the world gathered in San Francisco on March 13 and 14, 1981, to update and share their experience with health professionals.

The symposium was generously supported by the California Division of the American Cancer Society, Varian Associates, Ross Laboratories, Adria Laboratories, Atomic Energy of Canada Ltd., and Siemens Corporation.

Jerome M. Vaeth
President, West Coast Cancer Foundation

Front. Radiat. Ther. Onc., vol. 16, pp. 1–8 (Karger, Basel 1982)

Introduction

Stephen K. Carter

Northern California Cancer Program, Palo Alto, Calif., USA

Pediatric oncology is an area where combined modality therapy is required within a setting of expertise and adequate supportive care. Since the incidence of most pediatric tumors is not great, clinical research requires collaborative interaction and a proper interactive relationship with the community physician. If clinical research is to be successful, it requires that community pediatric physicians either participate in clinical research, or refer their patients to centers where clinical research is undertaken, whichever is appropiate.

The dual need in pediatric oncology is to maximize the resources for clinical research and to insure that every child diagnosed with malignancy receive the maximal benefit of existing knowledge and the resultant curative potential of therapy.

Pediatric malignancies differ from those of adults with respect to site, histopathology, clinical stage at diagnosis and other prognostic factors which are associated closely with outcome. Primary tumors in the lung, breast, gastrointestinal and genitourinary tract are rarely seen in children. The sites most frequently involved in the pediatric age group are the hematopoietic system, nervous system, muscles, bones and kidneys. Histologically, adenocarcinomas are uncommon in children so that the major histology in pediatric oncology is sarcoma. The majority of children are diagnosed with their malignancies at a late stage of clinical involvment. *Hammond* [3] has reviewed the frequency of pediatric cancers among 28 institutions in the Children's Cancer Study Group (table I). Leukemias accounted for 40% of the cancer diagnoses and lymphomas 10%. Cancers of the nervous system, including the brain, neuroblastoma and retinoblastoma, accounted for over

Table I. Percent distribution of the principle cancers of infants and children among 13, 601 patients registered by institutions participating in children's cancer study group 1974–1980

Disease	%	
Leukemia	40	
ALL/AUL		34
ANLL		5
Other leukemias		1
Lymphoma	10	
Hodgkin's		4
Non-Hodgkin's		6
Brain	10	
Neuroblastoma	8	
Retinoblastoma	3	
Bone	7	
Wilms'	6	
Rhabdomyosarcoma	5	
Others	11	

Derived from *Hammond* [3].

20% of the total. The remaining 30% are primarly cancers of the musculo-skeletal system and kidneys.

Pediatric solid tumors provide a model for the development of a successful treatment strategy. *Hammond* [3] has reviewed the milestones in this triumph over tragedy (table II).

The essence of a successful therapeutic attack against pediatric solid tumors involves a combination of local and metastatic control. Historically, successful therapy began with the local and regional control applications for surgery and X-ray. With the ability to achieve local and regional control, a study of relapse patterns showed the importance of metastatic control. Since many relapses after local control were metastatic, it became obvious that microscopic metastatic disease was present at the time of initial therapy. Fortunately, in pediatric tumors, drug responsiveness was observed early in the history of cytotoxic chemotherapy for cancer. The pediatric oncologists were among the first to recognize the potential value of adding drugs to surgery and/or X-ray in order to accomplish increased cure rates. The data in Wilms' tumors, Ewing's sarcoma and rhabdomyosarcoma have demonstrated

Table II. Ten milestones in the successful treatment of solid tumors of children

1	Extirpative surgery
2	Postoperative radiation therapy
3	Activity of single chemotherapeutic agents
4	Effective combinations of active agents
5	Combined modality therapy
6	Development of multidisciplinary therapy teams
7	Identification of new and refinement of prognostic variables
8	Development and refinement of systems of staging
9	Differential therapy approaches based on prognosis
	A Less aggressive therapy for patients with good prognosis
	B More aggressive therapy for patients with poor prognosis
10	Widespread application of new technologies

Derived from *Hammond* [3].

the validity of the concept. An example of the impact of successful combined therapy can be seen in the 2-year survival in Wilms' tumor from 1920 to 1975 in data published by *D'Angio and Belasko* [2] (table III).

Wilms' tumor provides an excellent model for the development of the successful multimodal approach. The first triumph was in pediatric surgery where the first cures were obtained in what had previously been a uniformly fatal disease. The early surgery had high mortality and low cure rates but importantly began the concept of treatment for cure. With improvement in anesthesiology and supportive care, the curative potential for surgery reached the 40% range and operative mortality dropped to below 5%. It was then found that Wilms' tumor was responsive to irradiation and the two modalities were combined to bring the cure rate up to 50%. Then came the discovery of chemotherapy with drugs such as actinomycin D and methotrexate being in the early forefront, soon to be followed by vincristine.

Out of all of this, came the landmark advance of the development of multidisciplinary teams. A great deal of the success in pediatric oncology can be ascribed to the appearance of these groups in specialized centers. Thus, permitting each child to obtain the benefit of expert consultations and care from the moment of diagnosis.

As the potential for multidisciplinary clinical research became evident, the low incidence of Wilms' tumor in any single institution made

Table III. Wilms' tumor survival

Year	Alive at 2 years[1], %
1920	8
1930	15
1940	32
1950	47
1965	81
1975	90

Derived from *D'Angio and Belasko* [2].
[1] Survival rate 1920–1960 from Boston Children's Hospital, and 1975 data from National Wilms' Tumor Study Group.

obvious the need for collaboration. As a result, cooperative clinical trial groups became the major focus for clinical research although a few institutions had enough patient material to pursue an individual course of research.

As the tumor became studied intensively, a staging system was evolved and the importance of clinical trials designed for individual subsets became obvious. The result was the formation of the first intergroup organization named the national Wilms' Tumor Study Group (NWTS). The NWTS has completed two studies (table IV).

These studies have established the following about the therapy of Wilms' tumor. (1) In group I disease, there is no need for postoperative irradiation in children who receive both actinomycin D and vincristine for at least 6 months. (2) In group II and III disease, the combination of actinomycin D and vincristine is superior to either agent used alone. (3) Adriamycin added to actinomycin D and vincristine is superior to the two drugs in groups II through IV.

As clinical research has been successfully developed and implemented, greater understanding of the disease itself has come about. For example, *Beckwith and Palmer* [1] have divided Wilms' tumor into favorable and unfavorable histology groups. In the NWTS-I, the unfavorable histology group accounted for only 11% of the 427 cases reviewed, but accounted for 43% of the deaths. The 2-year survival rates for the favorable and unfavorable histology were 89 and 39% respectively. The unfavorable group has been further subdivided into four subtypes: focal anaplasia; diffuse anaplasia; rhabdoid sarcoma,

Table IV. 2 year results of the NWTS

Study	Group or stage	Regimen	2-year survival, %	
			relapse-free	overall
NWTS-I	I	X-ray + actinomycin D	83	97
NWTS-II	I	actinomycin D + vincristine	85	95
NWTS-I	II+III	actinomycin D	57	67
		vincristine	55	72
		actinomycin D + vincristine	81	86
NWTS-II	II+III+IV	actinomycin D + vincristine	67	79
		same + adriamycin	80	86

NWTS grouping system
I   = Tumor limited to the kidney and completely excised
II = tumor extends beyond the kidney but is completely excised
III = Residual nonhematogenous tumor confined to abdomen
IV = Metastatic disease

and clear cell sarcoma. The rhabdoid sarcoma type is associated with both cerebral metastases and the appearance of independent second brain tumors arising in the posterior fossa. The clear cell sarcoma tends to metastasize to bone. This kind of detailed understanding of the heterogeneity within a disease process makes the necessity for collaborative clinical research even more imperative.

As clinical research becomes successful in a tumor, it can be expected that prognostic factors will shift in importance. In addition, differential strategies will be required for those at high risk for therapeutic failure as against those at low risk. The third protocol of the NWTS now divides the patients into favorable and unfavorable histology groups and asks different questions in both.

Successful therapy changes some of the considerations in clinical research. When it is possible to cure a large percentage of patients then a research thrust to diminish the morbidity and mortality of therapy becomes both logical and feasible. This has begun to occur in pediatric oncology to a significant degree and will hopefully provide a viable model for adult oncology. The diminishment of treatment-related morbidity is occurring along two broad lines, within a combined modality approach to pediatric solid tumors. One thrust is to diminish the intensity of the systemic drug treatment. This involves utilizing less drugs or a shorter duration of therapy. An example can be seen in the current third study of NWTS. In stage I patients, they are testing whether the results with 10 weeks of actinomycin D and vincristine are comparable to the use of both agents for 6 months. In stage II patients, NWTS-3 is asking whether routine postoperative radiation of the flank is necessary in patients receiving effective chemotherapy.

A second approach is to diminish the intensity of local control therapy since effective systemic therapy can be counted upon. This can result in less functional impairment from surgery or less long-term complications from intensive irradiation. An example of this approach is in osteogenic sarcoma where the use of aggressive drug treatment has enabled surgical resection and endoprosthetic replacement to be utilized instead of radical amputation. *Rosen* [4] demonstrated the effectiveness of this approach in lesions of both the lower and upper extremities. In his studies, histologic review of multiple sections taken from the specimens resected following preoperative chemotherapy have revealed varying degrees of tumor necrosis attributable to the drug treatment.

The majority of patients so treated had greater than 90% tumor necrosis within the entire resected specimen. All of these patients have remained disease-free. In the Memorial Hospital series, ten metastatic relapses have occurred and, in all, the effect of preoperative chemotherapy on the primary tumor had been less than 90% tumor necrosis.

The current study at Memorial Hospital calls for preoperative weekly high-dose methotrexate with citrovorum factor rescue. Patients with lesions in the proximal humerus have surgery following 4 weeks of therapy, with patients awaiting the custom-production of an endoprosthesis for lesions of the distal femur have 16 weeks of preoperative chemotherapy with the addition of BCD (bleomycin, cyclophosphamide and actinomycin D) and adriamycin cyclically. Following resection, the entire specimen is examined by a single pathologist and the effect of drug treatment determined. Those patients deemed to have less than 90% tumor necrosis are assigned to an alternate postoperative chemotherapy regimen containing high dose cis-platinum in combination with adriamycin, as well as the BCD triple regimen. The patients

Table V. The multidisciplinary management team

Primary physician	Nurse
Radiologist	Pharmacologist
Pathologist	Clinical Pharmacist
Biochemist	Microbiologist
Immunologist	Nutritionist
Surgeon	Rehabilitationist
Chemotherapist	Psychologist
Radiation Therapist	Social Worker

who have a complete or near complete effect of preoperative chemotherapy on the primary tumor continue on the same chemotherapy with an attempt being made to reduce the duration of treatment needed to achieve disease-free suvival. To date, 69 of 71 patients treated on this protocol remain disease-free. This includes 24 of 26 with poor response to the preoperative regimen and switched to the alternative aggressive multidrug combination.

From an overall perspective, the triumph of pediatric oncology today is a triumph of the multidisciplinary management concept. The advances have resultedt from collaboration among the medical disciplines involved in the diagnoisis and treatment of cancer. The majority of children diagnosed with cancer in the United States are managed not by one specialist after another, but by teams that have been developed in the nation's major pediatric referral institutions. The variety of disciplines required for the sophisticated management of infants and children with cancer are listed in table V.

The trained personnel, facilities, equipment and other resources needed to provide the best available treatment for the cancers cannot be developed in most of the nation's community hospitals. Given the relative rarity of these tumors, their care may be more appropriately the mission of a pediatric medical center providing tertiary care. However, as *Hammond* [3] points out, centers capable of providing state-of-the-art pediatric cancer management are having a significant nationwide impact on the management of children through cancer control programs. This makes pediatric oncologic specialists, their expertise and their institutional facilities more widely known and available to the professionals involved in the medical care of children in their region.

This symposium covers the entire range of triumphs in pediatric oncology including the implications of successful therapy for future research. This includes the delayed toxicities of chemotherapy on childhood tissues, as discussed by Dr. *Bleyer* and of radiation therapy as addressed by Dr. *Rubin.* In addition, Dr. *Donaldson* presents data on Hodgkin's disease and the reduction of the radiotherapy dose. The symposium also gives proper emphasis to the multidisciplinary approach to care that is required. This includes 'the cancer unit' as outlined by Dr. *Wilbur,* nursing care [*Lorraine Bivalec*], the impact of cancer on the family [Dr. *Spinetta*], the pharmacist's view of drug testing for children [Dr. *Glaubiger*] and the nutrition of children with cancer [Dr. *Van Eys*].

References

1   Beckwith, J.B.; Palmer, N.F: Histopathology and prognosis of Wilms' tumor – results from the First National Wilm's Tumor Study. Cancer *41:* 1937–1948 (1978).
2   D'Angio, G.J., Belasko, J.B.: Wilms' Tumor; in Burchenal, Oettgen, Cancer – achievements, challenges and prospects for the 1980s, pp. 191–201 (Grune & Stratton, New York 1981).
3   Hammond, H.: in Burchenal, Oettgen, Cancer – Achievements, challenges and prospects for the 1980s (Grune & Stratton, New York 1981).
4   Rosen, G.: Current management of malignant bone sarcoma; in Burchenal, Oettgen, Cancer – achievement, challenges and prospects for the 1980s, pp. 213–223 1(Grune & Stratton, New York 1981.

S.K. Carter, MD, Director, Northern California Cancer Program,
Palo Alto, CA 94304 (USA)

Front. Radiat. Ther. Onc., vol. 16, pp. 9–17 (Karger, Basel 1982)

Epidemiologic Characteristics of Childhood Cancer[1]

Donald F. Austin, Verne E. Nelson, Linda F. Johnson

Resource for Cancer Epidemiology, Health Services, Oakland, Calif., USA

The title 'Triumph Over Tragedy' is an unusual topic for a conference on cancer. The war on cancer is generally fought on two broad fronts: that of prevention and that of treatment. There is little to talk about in the area of prevention of childhood cancer, but in the area of treatment there have been some dramatic improvements. For example, the average time from diagnosis to death for a child diagnosed with leukemia was, in the 1940s and early 1950s, commonly about 6 weeks. In the 1960s, that prognosis became about 6 months, and in the 1970s about 5–6 years. In the 1980s, the term 'cure' is now being used.

It seems fashionable today to challenge the validity of any claim of success in the field of cancer and the apparent success in therapy of childhood cancer is no exception. The best illustration is the controversy over chemotherapy in osteogenic sarcoma [2]. There are at least two alternative arguments offered for an apparent increase in survival rate with chemotherapy in this disease.

The first argument is that there is really an improvement, but it is due to an improvement in surgery, not in chemotherapy. The second argument is that there is really no improvement in survival, but that the apparent improvement is due to better staging and to a changing pattern of referral to major treatment centers from which most treatment data come. Most conclusions of treatment improvements are based on clinical trials and there is no substitute for clinical trials for this purpose. Therefore, epidemiologists seldom become involved. However, in this instance, epidemiology can be useful in examining the validity

[1] This project was partially supported by NCI contract No. NO1 CP-81018.

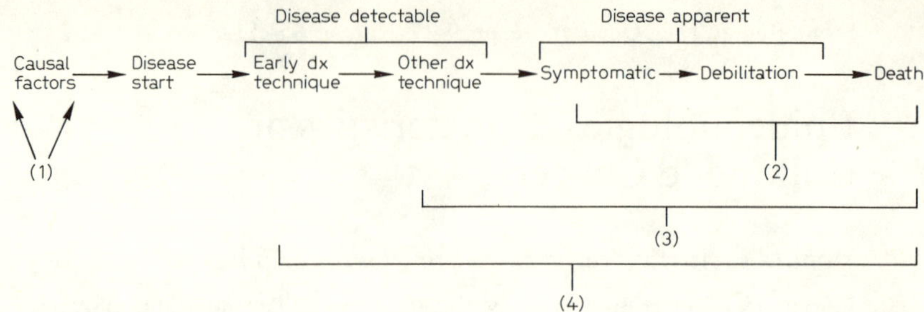

Fig. 1. General stages in the progression of a malignancy. 1 = Prevention; 2 = survival time with 'late' diagnosis; 3 = survival time with average diagnosis; 4 = survival time with 'early' diagnosis.

of the second alternative explanation: i.e., that there really is no improvement in survival in childhood cancer in general, or for specific sites.

Figure 1 is a schematic representation of the stages of progression of a malignancy from its start, without treatment, to death of the patient. It illustrates one basic point about survival rates: namely, that they are based on an observation period which has its end at the point of death and its start at the point of diagnosis. As one progresses from point 2 to point 3 to point 4 in this diagram, one can see that the observation period becomes longer and longer, thus creating longer survival rates for those individuals diagnosed at points 2, 3 and 4, but with no actual length in life. One explanation for the apparent increase in survival with chemotherapy patients is our increased ability to diagnose at an earlier stage and to place patients more accurately into the correct points along the schematic diagram. The second explanation for an improvement in survival rates is a proposed increasing proportion of patients referred to treatment centers who are in the early stages of their disease, thus creating a group of patients with a very favorable prognosis when compared to past patients.

One statistic that cannot be affected by these factors is the mortality rate. It is, therefore, pertinent to determine whether the mortality from childhood cancer is really declining.

Figure 2 shows childhood cancer mortality rates for California in 1950 [3], in 1960, in 1969–1971 and in 1976–1978 [4, 5]. It is apparent that, in each 5-year age-group or in all childhood groups combined, cancer mortality rates have declined substantially. From a high of approximately 400 deaths per 1,000,000 in 1950, there were approxi-

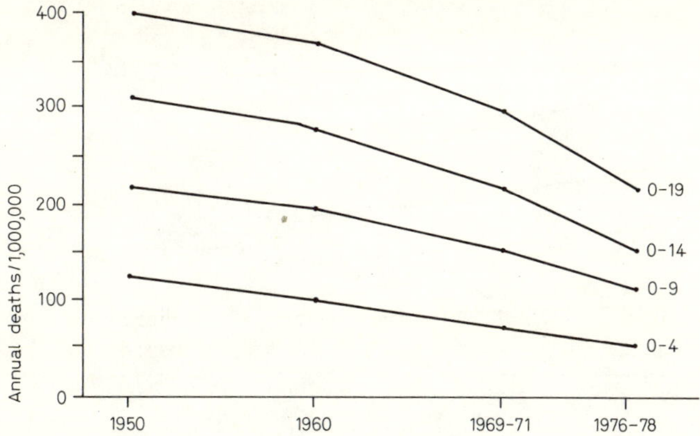

Fig. 2. California childhood cancer mortality rates, 1950–1978 [from ref. 3–5].

Table I. Distribution of newly diagnosed childhood cancer (0–19 years) by site, SF-O SMSA, 1969–1978 (n = 1,518) [6]

Site	Percent
Acute leukemia	20.7
Brain	15.7
Hodgkin's disease	10.0
Bone	5.9
Non-Hodgkin's lymphoma	5.9
Soft tissue	4.9
Kidney	4.3
Thyroid	3.6
Melanoma of skin	3.0
Eye	2.8
Testis	2.4
All other sites	19.6

mately 250 deaths per 1,000,000 in the period 1976–1978. Also, note that the decline in mortality rates for the last 5-year age-group shown, i.e., ages 15–19, seems less than those of other age-groups.

The major types of cancer of all childhood malignancies are made up of acute leukemia, brain tumors, Hodgkin's and non-Hodgkin's lymphomas and sarcomas, including both bone and soft-tissue sarcomas (table I). Grouped together, those form about two-thirds of all childhood tumors up to the age of 19. The distribution of childhood

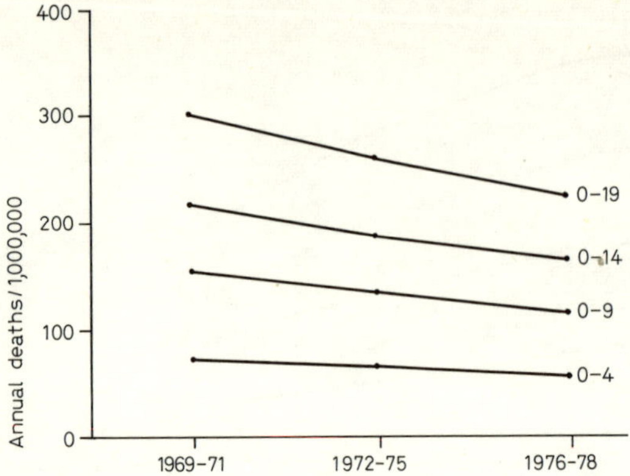

Fig. 3. Cumulative mortality rates for cancer in childhood (0–19 years) for California [from ref. 4, 5].

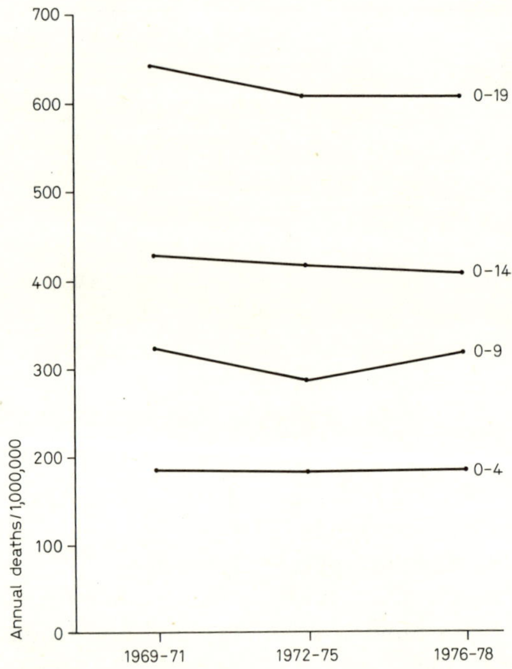

Fig. 4. Cumulative incidence rates for cancer in childhood (0–19 years) SF-O SMSA [from ref. 6].

Table II. Mortality/incidence index for childhood cancer by 5-year age-group, 1969–1978 (California cancer death rates divided by SF-O SMSA cancer incidence rates × 100) [6]

	Age-group				
3-year period	0–4	5–9	10–14	15–19	0–19
1969–1971	40	60	60	39	48
1970–1972	35	67	52	41	46
1971–1973	33	66	46	40	44
1972–1974	37	69	41	40	44
1973–1975	38	62	42	36	43
1974–1976	36	57	50	39	44
1975–1977	31	54	49	36	40
1976–1978	31	43	46	35	38

tumors up through age 14 has fewer female genital and thyroid cancers and proportionally more acute leukemias, but the relative ranking of these major tumors remains the same.

Figure 3 shows in more detail the mortality rate for childhood cancer by 5–year age-groups for the 10-year period 1969–78. Here again, it is apparent that mortality rates for each childhood age-group are decreasing. This decrease could occur in several ways other than from an improvement in therapy; for example, the incidence of childhood cancer could be decreasing. However, the incidence, figure 4, as measured by the incidence rates for the five Bay Area counties, is remaining essentially the same [6]. And, when comparing the mortality and incidence data, there appears to be, for each age-group, a widening difference between incidence and mortality. It is also apparent from these two figures that for each age-group the mortality rate in 1976–78 is less than half of the incidence rate. This means that for every 100 cases that occur there are fewer than 50 deaths. This is not equivalent to saying that out of every 100 patients diagnosed there will be fewer than 50 deaths. Rather, it is analogous to saying that for every 100 apples, there are 50 oranges which, of course, is different from implying that out of every 100 apples, 50 will become oranges. This mortality/incidence index, even though it does not imply that the deaths occurring in a single year come from among those cases who are diagnosed in that year, is nevertheless a very sensitive index of the status of medical therapy.

Table III. Mortality/incidence index[1] for childhood cancers, 1969–1978, malignancy type [6]

Time period	Leukemia[2]	Brain[2]	Bone[2]	Connective and soft tissue
1969–1971	83	38	56	42
1972–1975	63	40	46	19
1976–1978	70	24	38	29

[1] California cancer mortality rates divided by SF-O SMSA cancer incidence rates for children, 0–19, age-adjusted.
[2] Significant ($p < 0.05$) decreases in mortality over 1969–1978 period, based on test of slope for simple linear regression.

Table IV. Mortality/incidence index for childhood leukemia in the SF-O SMSA, by age-group (1973–1977) [6]

Age	0–4	5–9	0–14	15–19
Index	21	65	74	86

Table II shows the mortality/incidence index for childhood cancer over a 10-year period in California. The index is simply the California mortality rate divided by the incidence rate for five Bay Area counties in California. One can see from the top figure in the first column, which is 40, that for each 100 cases of childhood cancer diagnosed in the 0–4 age-group, there are 40 deaths. If each of the first four columns is examined, there appears a definite (and in most columns quite large) decrease in the index, indicating marked improvement in therapy. Those who claim that we are not really curing cases of childhood cancer but are, rather, postponing their deaths to a later time period, might find some support from the data presented in this table. For example, in the first three figures in the first column, there exists a sizable decrease in the index. In the 5–9 age-group, the second column, an almost exactly compensating increase exists. Similar examples may be found in this table. Because of that, the 15–19 age-group is included. In that age-group there seems to be only a slight decrease. Higher age-groups do not show increases. Even when all age-groups up through age 19 are combined, a definite overall decrease of approximately 20% over the 10-year period is apparent.

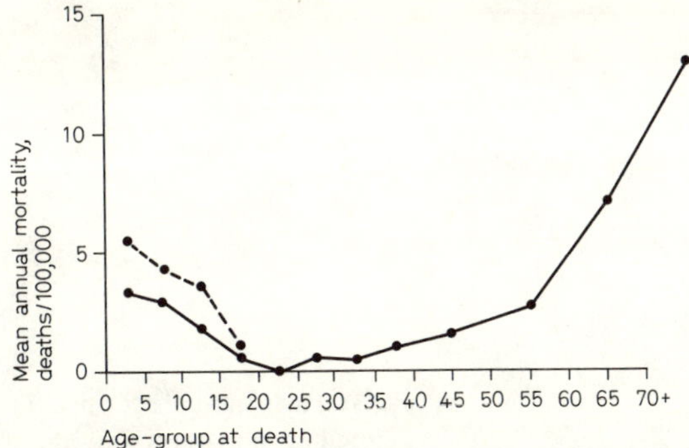

Fig. 5. Mean annual age-specific acute leukemia mortality rates, Buffalo, N.Y., 1959–1961 [from ref. 6; raw data supplied by *Warren Winkelstein, Jr.,* University of California School of Public Health, Berkeley]. – – – = Total leukemia; ———— = acute leukemia.

Table III shows the mortality/incidence index for some of the more common childhood cancers for the same time period: leukemia, brain, bone and connective and soft tissue. In each one of these categories, a decrease exists. What appears to be surprising is the fact that the index is so high for leukemia. One might anticipate figures less than 50% for leukemia, based on the index for all cancers. This apparent discrepancy stems from the widely different 5-year age-group indices for leukemia (table IV). Although the index in the 0–4 group is very low, approximately one death for every 5 cases diagnosed, in the 15–19 age-group, nearly nine deaths occur for every 10 cases diagnosed. The difference in the prognosis for children in their late teens as compared to the first 5 years of life is so great that when all age-groups are combined, the total mortality/incidence index is rather high. This difference is intriguing for another reason: here is a biological response to therapy which parallels an occurrence pattern for leukemia.

Figure 5 illustrates the age-specific mortality for leukemia through ages 0–70+. Because these data were taken from 1960, they are very similar to incidence rates. This figure illustrates a characteristic and unique pattern for leukemia, e.g., that acute leukemia increases in adult life with an ever-increasing rate beginning at about the age of 20. This pattern is fairly characteristic for the results of cumulative effects and has been interpreted to represent, for acute leukemia, the cumulative effects of environmental insults such as exposures to radiation or organic solvents. In contrast, the curve during childhood is one of a

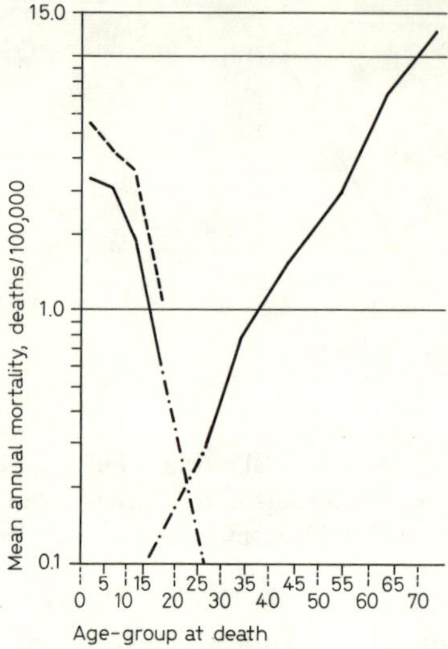

Fig. 6. Mean annual age-specific acute leukemia mortality rates, Buffalo, N.Y., 1959–1961, with projected adult and childhood patterns [from ref. 6; raw data. Supplied by *Warren Winkelstein, Jr.,* University of California School of Public Health, Berkeley]. – – – = Total leukemia; ——— = acute leukemia; –·– = projected.

decreasing rate, reaching the lowest point at about age 25. This pattern is more reminiscent of the last or descending portion of a typical epidemic curve. If so, this would suggest exposures in the very early period, such as prenatal exposures.

It is possible to examine the slopes of those curves on a logarithmic scale, which better illustrates rates of change. Figure 6 shows that the rate of increase for adult leukemia is fairly constant; and, if one projects that line to its approximate origin, one finds that it may originate in the mid-teens. Conversely, the line for childhood leukemia illustrates a fairly constant rate of decrease, which if projected to its approximate completion, suggests a termination in the mid-twenties. These two intersecting lines suggest that cases diagnosed between the approximate ages of 15–25 are a mixture of the two types of diseases. These two occurrence patterns suggest two etiologically different diseases. Their response to therapy suggests two biologically different diseases. The response to therapy for patients first diagnosed in the late teens, suggests that many of these patients belong to the adult biological type of leukemia.

There is not a lot known as to the causes of childhood leukemia. Prenatal irradiation is known to be a cause, but other than certain chromosomal abnormalities which apparently predispose to leukemia, little is certain about the cause or causes of childhood leukemia. Viruses, because of their relationship to certain animal leukemias, have always been suspect. Several years ago, we reported the finding that children born of mothers who were in their first trimester of pregnancy coincident with an influenza A epidemic, had a three- to four-fold risk of childhood leukemia [1]. No one would suggest that influenza A is a leukemogenic virus, but it has been suggested that certain antigenic stimuli to the fetus at a critical time in its development by certain biological agents such as influenza A might create a population of white cells peculiarly susceptible to leukemia. Clusters of childhood leukemia cases have been investigated almost uniformly without usefull knowledge resulting. The usual conclusion of the investigation of childhood leukemia clusters has been that they represented instances of very rare phenomena occurring very rarely.

Childhood leukemia is not the only childhood malignancy which may occur in clusters. Ewing's sarcoma, a very uncommon bone cancer, may sometimes occur in clusters. For example, in the 3-million population that we monitor, there have been 30 recorded cases in an 8-year period. 20% of the entire 8-year incidence occur in one small community, within a 30-block diameter. Clusters such as these are so dramatic that they demand investigation. Our hope is that these investigations may bring some clues as to how to prevent the disease so that we can bring a degree of success in the area of prevention of childhood cancer to match the present triumph in its treatment.

References

1   Austin, D.; Karp, S.; Dworsky, R.; Henderson, B.: Excess leukemia in cohorts of children born following influenza epidemics. Am. J. Epidem. *101:*77–83 (1975).
2   Kolata, G.B.: Dilemma in cancer treatment. Science *209:*792–794 (1980).
3   Schoen, R.; Collins, M.: Mortality by cause: life tables for California, 1950–1970. Calif. State Dept of Public Health (1973).
4   State of California. Dept of Health Services: Vital statistics of California, 1970–1978 (forthcoming).
5   State of California. Dept of Finance: Population projections for California counties 1975–2020. Rep. 77-P-3 (1977).
6   State of California. Dept of Health Services: Resource for cancer epidemiology. Cancer Incidence System. Database records, 1969–1978.

D.F. Austin, MD, Resource for Cancer Epidemiology, Health Services,
1450 Broadway, Oakland, CA 94612 (USA)

Front. Radiat. Ther. Onc., vol. 16, pp. 18–29 (Karger, Basel 1982)

Leukemia: Historical Development of Cancer Therapy

The First Battle is Won[1]

Audrey E. Evans

Children's Hospital of Philadelphia, Cancer Center, Division of Oncology,
University of Pennsylvania, Philadelphia, Pa., USA

Introduction

This paper attempts to show how the treatment of leukemia in childhood evolved over the past 4 decades, how initial successes in the 40s led to carefully designed studies to improve on the results so that finally at the end of the 70s the goal was reached, that is, cure of childhood acute lymphocytic leukemia (ALL). These have become the prototype for many other clinical studies of cancer in both children and adults. Pediatric oncologists are to be congratulated for their willingness to collaborate with others in the same and different disciplines to mount an all-out attack on what was initially a hopeless disease. However, cure of only some children with leukemia is still not enough, the pediatrician aims at cure of all. Moreover, the heritage of pediatrics is the prevention of disease. The ultimate battle thus will be won only when methods are found to prevent leukemia, which – in this context – can be viewed as a disorder of cellular maturation.

Each decade had differing goals and the tempo of research accelerated rapidly as each new discovery was made. A larger proportion of the work was devoted to study of ALL. Acute myeloid leukemia tended to take second place, in part because the incidence was less and because treatment was less effective.

[1] Supported by NIH grant Nos CA-19372, CA-14489 and CA-11796.

1940–1949: The Search for a Treatment

The initial therapy for leukemia was with irradiation. Attempts to use this mode of treatment were made almost immediately after the discovery of the miraculous X-ray and radium. Indeed, the concept that systemic treatment was needed is implicit in *Dessauer's* proposal in 1905 [3] that total body irradiation should be employed. Splenic irradiation and treatment of enlarged nodes had already been used, and continued to be the usual technique. In 1924, *Minot* et al. [21] were able to report better results in 78 patients irradiated for chronic myelogenous leukemia, than for their 52 nonirradiated cohorts. They stated in a subsequent report that irradiation results were better in those with myelogenous rather than lymphatic leukemias, especially in children, who seemed to be made worse. It is of interest that they measured benefit as improvement in the quality of life, because they found that survival time was not prolonged, a prescient observation that was to be reported by others using different treatments later in the century. In the 1940s alkylating agents were being developed. Nitrogen mustard caused transient falls in blast cell counts and decreased the size of enlarged lymph nodes [13].

The major breakthrough came in 1948 when *Farber* et al. [4] at the Children's Hospital in Boston reported temporary remissions lasting a few months in 10 out of 16 leukemic children following therapy with the folic acid antagonist, aminopterin. This signal advance is itself an example of the systematic, step-by-step progress that happily has characterized pediatric oncologic research. First, it was reasoned that the newly identified hematopoietic maturation factor, folic acid, might have a similar effect on leukemic cells. It was tried in the clinic – and here there was a happy coincidence of an alert physician and a serendipitous occurrence. Postmortem studies of leukemic infiltrates of the bone marrow and viscera in patients treated with folic acid conjugates were regarded by *Farber* et al. [4] as evidence of an acceleration of the process, not a slowing. The extent of leukemic involvement was more than encountered before then in some 200 postmortem examinations of children with leukemia. Then why not try the reverse? A series of folic acid antagonists were synthesized specifically for that purpose by *Subbarow*. Starting treatment in November 1947, with intramuscular aminopterin, several children had clearing of blasts from their bone marrows and regeneration of normal marrow cells.

These early results stimulated a search for other agents that would act as antimetabolites. Preliminary trials with hormones such as prednisone [23] and ACTH [5] were also under way and were found to produce transient normalization of peripheral counts and bone marrow. Thus, in this decade agents had been found which could induce remissions of leukemia.

1950–1959: Increasing the Remission Rate

Early in the 50s came the discovery and clinical use of purine antagonists; 6MP [1] was the most successful of these analogues. Research emphasis continued to be placed on the discovery of new agents capable of inducing remissions, but treatment by and large continued to be with single agent chemotherapy. A remission was induced and maintained as long as possible before the inevitable relapse when a second and third agent was introduced. There were attempts to use the agents more effectively by dose and schedule though bone marrow and other organ toxicity limited the doses of everything but corticosteroids.

The induction rate of most of the agents used alone was in the order of 30%. Later in the decade, methotrexate or 6MP were used in conjunction with prednisone and a significant increase in the remission rate resulted. Attention by then also was being given to some of the complications of leukemia such as central nervous system infiltration and measures were designed to treat meningeal leukemia. Radiation therapy was used in modest doses and was found to be effective as was the intrathecal administration of chemotherapy [2, 29].

Treatment during this decade increased the median survival time of children with ALL from 4 to about 10 months and there were rare long-term survivors. There was, however, very little effective treatment for non-lymphocytic leukemia during this period.

Supportive care played its role with the increased use of blood products, in particular platelet concentrates which were effective in preventing bleeding in most cases. Antibiotics against gram-positive and gram-negative organisms also played a significant role in decreasing the number of infectious deaths during the initial period of treatment.

The new antileukemic agents being developed through this decade required tests for anti-leukemic activity and needed to be compared with more established drugs. Groups of investigators joined together to form cooperative groups so that clinical trials could be conducted to answer these questions. Two of the groups have recently celebrated their 25th anniversaries, the Children's Cancer Study Group and Acute Leukemia Group B, now known as Cancer and Acute Leukemia Group B. In this way research could be accelerated and meaningful comparisons made with large numbers of patients.

1960–1969: Prolongation of Remission and Attempts at Cure

During this decade clinical research accelerated greatly. The co-operative groups created in the 50s carried out a series of randomized comparative clinical trials. Combinations of chemotherapy were given to induce remissions and rates increased to 80% in certain groups of patients [22]. Focus was placed on the prevention of relapse, and the word 'cure' began to be used. Phases of therapy were designed and termed 'induction', 'consolidation' and 'maintenance', the aim being to prevent the development of resistant cells which could lead to relapse. The 'total therapy' series of clinical trials for leukemia at St. Jude Children's Research Hospital led by *Pinkel*, started during this period; cure of leukemia was their bold goal [8]. Innovative investigations were designed at the National Cancer Institute (NCI) to maintain 'pharmacologic pressure', introducing drugs into treatment schedules at times when theoretically the burden of leukemic cells was at its lowest. Much of this work was based on the studies of *Skipper* et al. [25] who were able to show by means of a mouse leukemia model that drugs reduce cell populations proportionally dose-for-dose and that cells regrow steadily in similar fashion when they escape chemotherapy control. Treatment regimens containing multiple drugs in use at the NCI during this period had the acronyms VAMP [6] and POMP [11]. These efforts did indeed prolong the remission duration considerably, but did not significantly increase the number of patients who were cured – shades of Minot. This was also the era when the cyclic use of multiple agents was put to the test, as in the BIKE NCI regimen [7] and the one used by *Zeulzer* [30]. He employed chemotherapy in 6-week cycles to see if several agents used in such fashion were more effective than when they were used in the more conventional way, that is singly until relapse. A study by the Children's Cancer Study Group comparing 'cyclic' versus 'sequential' treatment showed that the cycles as planned did not significantly prolong the overall survival [15].

During this period, attention was directed to the so-called 'sanctuary' sites, the central nervous system being the most important one. In the latter part of the 60s, regimens included treatment of the central nervous system with irradiation, chemotherapy or both before there was gross evidence of meningeal involvement. *Mathe* et al. [16] found in a review of biopsy material that numerous sites such as the liver, kidney and central nervous system of patients in what seemed to be hematologic remission often harbored leukemic cells in these sanctuary sites. A study in Minnesota was designed, therefore, to test the use of low-dose irradiation to some of the sanctuary areas including the liver and kidneys. Percutaneous biopsies taken before and after therapy showed clearing of these sites [14].

Other attempts to improve remission duration were made with nonspecific immunotherapy such as BCG or C Parvum. This approach seemed at first to be promising, but subsequent studies were not able to show a benefit from nonspecific immune stimulation [12, 17, 19].

Meanwhile, irradiation was being used in major ways. Extracorporeal irradiation to reduce the number of circulating leukemic cells was tried and bone marrow transplantation incorporating total body irradiation came of age during this period [26]. New information on tissue typing led the way for successful transplantation of normal bone marrow cells from a matched related donor. The early attempts were made mostly in patients with far advanced disease, and many of them succumbed to various complications let alone recurrence of the leukemic process. There were, however, some long-term survivors, suggesting that the method had promise for the cure of patients with leukemia. Autologous bone marrow harvested when the patient was in remission and reinfused later, also was attempted at this time. This technique permitted the delivery of treatment to induce another remission, but its obvious disadvantage was the possibility that the stored specimen contained leukemic cells. This method did not lead to a large proportion of long-term survivors.

1970–1979: Cure is Achieved

The several efforts made during the 60s reached fruition in the 70s when several studies of combined treatment for ALL reported many long-term survivors. The therapy used in these endeavors included the knowledge generated during the 60s regarding the best agents for induction, the need for consolidation including attention to sanctuary sites, and need for continuing therapy in order to maintain remission. By the middle of the 70s it was found that more than 50% of the children with ALL were surviving and in continuous remission for 5 years [9]. Those who relapsed did so during the first 2 or 2½ years and few thereafter. At this time trials were designed to determine how long treatment should be continued. Patients were treated for 2½ or 3 years and then randomized to stop or continue therapy until 5 or 6 years. It was found that continuing chemotherapy beyond 2½ or 3 years did not improve the survival rate except in boys who have a tendency to develop testicular relapses [24].

One of the major contributions of the cooperative groups during this period, and in particular, the Children's Cancer Study Group, was the study of 'natural history' factors. Physical findings and laboratory data present at diagnosis were analyzed to determine which features had prognostic value. It has long been known that older age, high WBC, central nervous system involvement, and a mediastinal mass affected the prognosis adversely. The large numbers of patients treated on a uniform protocol allowed analysis of many more prognostic factors, their relative importance and their interrelationship one with another. Essentially this is 'staging' of the disease as in any form of cancer.

Leukemia staging has achieved sufficient precision that it can now be used to design treatment regimens tailored to the prognosis [20]. To some extent prognostic factors vary in importance depending upon the end point being analyzed; for example, those affecting remission induction are not the same as those associated with remission duration or survival, although the height of the initial WBC is important for all of them. Several new items were included in this study of prognostic factors; among them lymphoblast morphology according to the FAB classification, histological stains such as PAS and Sudan Black, serum immunoglobulins, B and T cell markers and HLA typing. Not all were found to have prognostic import. Table I lists the unfavorable prognostic factors when successful remission induction is the criterion.

Table II shows the predictors of disease-free survival by multivariate analysis together with the levels of statistical significance. The following factors define patients with an unfavorable outlook: $WBC > 20 \times 10^9/l$, hemoglobin greater than 10 g/dl, depressed immu-

Table I. Unfavorable prognostic factors of response to induction therapy; the prognostic significance of physical signs and laboratory data present at diagnosis on the remission induction rate of children with ALL [from ref. 9]

Factor	n*	Failure rate, %	p
Initial WBC $20 \times 10^9/1$	27/290	9.3	0.09
Age >10 years	23/200	11.5	0.01
40% PAS + blasts	21/154	13.6	0.007
Decreased IgG	11/113	9.7	0.009
L_2 morphology	8/85	9.41	0.0001
L_3 morphology	2/6	33.0	0.0001
M_3 marrow day 14	16/73	21.9	0.001
CNS disease at diagnosis	5/33	15.1	0.0001
Down's syndrome	2/15	13.3	0.09
Overall	49/880	5.6	

* Denominator = number of patients with the factor. Numerator = number of patients failing to achieve remission.

noglobulins, enlarged spleen, age under 2 and over 9 years, bone marrow not cleared of blasts after 14 days of treatment, male sex and L_2, L_3 morphology. It is interesting to note that some of the factors important for predicting successful induction, such as CNS disease at diagnosis, nodal and other organ enlargement, mediastinal mass, and race are no longer significant predictors of disease-free survival. Analysis of the data pin-pointed a so-called 'lymphoma syndrome' because it suggests progression of non-Hodgkin's lymphoma into the leukemic phase rather than leukemia arising de novo in the bone marrow. The lymphoma syndrome requires the presence of three or more of the following features: hemoglobin greater than 10 g, markedly enlarged liver, spleen or lymph nodes and a mediastinal mass.

These numerous subdivisions make it possible to divide patients into three prognostic groups designated good, average and poor. Children's Cancer Study Group protocols during the past 5 years have been designed differently for each of these three groups. Table III shows how patients are subdivided by white count, age, tumor burden and morphology. Since the majority of patients have null cell leukemia, the presence of B or T markers on the blasts did not have a strong effect on prognosis. Most often T cell leukemia is considered to have a bad prognosis mainly because of its association with an older

Table II. Predictors of disease-free survival by multivariate analysis; the importance of various prognostic indicators according to their level of significance and influence on the disease-free survival of children with ALL [9]

Rank	Variable	Significance level* (p value)
1	log WBC	0.002
2	hemoglobin	0.005
3	IgM	0.005
4	splenomegaly	0.007
5	age and age^2	0.04 and 0.014
6	day-14 marrow	0.03
7	sex	0.04
8	IgG	0.07
9	morphology	0.09

* Platelet count, CNS disease at diagnosis, nodal enlargement, mediastinal mass, race, and hepatomegaly were not significant predictors of outcome.

Table III. Newly defined prognostic groups determined by multivariate analysis of factors in CCG 141

Factor	Prognostic group		
	good[1]	average	poor[2]
WBC × 10^9/l	<20	20–100	>100[3]
Age, years	2–10	>10	<1
Lymphoma syndrome[3]	(0)	(<3)	(3 or more)
Hgb, g/dl	<10		$\geq$10
Liver, spleen, nodes	not markedly enlarged		markedly enlarged
Mediastinal mass	absent		present
CNS disease at diagnosis	absent	absent	present
FAB morphology	$\geq$ 75% L$_1$	$\geq$ 75% L$_1$	$\geq$ 25% L$_2$
Ig, depressed	0–1	0–3	0–3
Day-14 marrow	M$_1$ or M$_2$	M$_{1,2,3}$	M$_{1,2,3}$

[1] Good prognostic group: all features must be present.
[2] Poor prognostic group defined by presence of any one of the factors.
[3] Lymphoma syndrome defined by presence of 3 or more of the following features: Hgb >10 g/dl, markedly enlarged liver, spleen (below the umbilicus), and lymph nodes (>3 cm diameter or visible), and mediastinal mass.

boy, a mediastinal mass and a high white count. If these are not present, T cell marker per se, is not a bad prognostic factor [10].

With these well-defined prognostic factors, it is now possible to consider seriously the amount of treatment that needs be given each child. The disease-free survival of the good prognosis patient is now 90% at 5 years and it is reasonable to believe that an equally good result could be achieved with less aggressive therapy [20]. One of the areas that requires study is the best method for preventing central nervous system relapse, since the commonly used regimen of 2,400 rad of cranial irradiation with intrathecal and systemic methotrexate can be expected to cause future learning problems in some children according to studies at the Children's Hospital of Philadelphia [18].

Another innovative treatment introduced during the 70s was immunotherapy. This followed the initial work of *Mathe* et al. [16, 17] with BCG in the 60s. BCG and the MER preparations were employed in combination with chemotherapy both for lymphocytic and myeloid leukemia. Vaccines of leukemic cells were also tried as a more specific stimulant of the immune system. More recently the value of interferon is being explored to see whether some different manipulation of the immune system will be successful.

Nonlymphocytic Leukemia

Most of the foregoing relates to the treatment of childhood ALL. The pediatric oncologists together with their colleagues in adult cancer treatment struggled with the more resistant diseases of acute myeloid, promyelocytic and monocytic leukemia. The induction of remission with multiple agents including cytosine arabinoside, a purine antagonist and an anthracycline has increased the remission rate to about 70%, but maintenance treatment has not greatly prolonged the survival time nor led to many long-term survivors. However, there has been one major advance in the treatment of nonlymphocytic leukemia, and that is high-dose chemotherapy and total body irradiation followed by bone marrow transplantation from an HLA-identical sibling. (It is interesting to note in passing that, three quarters of a century later, we have returned to *Dessauer's* concepts [3] of total body irradiation for leukemia.) This is now considered in many centers to be the primary treatment during first remission and has led to a 2-year survival rate of 60% [27]. The results are not so good if the transplant is done while the patient is in relapse. In addition to BMT for acute nonlymphocytic leukemia there are some interesting data from a study at the Sidney Farber Cancer Center following aggressive treatment with cytosine arabinoside, adriamycin, vincristine, azacytidine, methotrexate and 6MP in various combinations for 1 year which may be leading to a significant increase in the number of long-term survivors [28].

Late Effects of Treatment

The study of the late effects of therapy came to the forefront in the latter part of the 70s with the increasing number of children who are surviving disease-free. The triumph would indeed be hollow if treatment cured children with leukemia, but left them permanently incapacitated.

The side effects of irradiation on growing and developing tissues of childhood are well known, but less obvious are those following chemotherapy. The vulnerable tissues which must be watched are the brain, pituitary gland, thyroid, heart, lung, liver, kidneys, ovaries, testes and spine. In the 60s there were reports of liver and cerebral dysfunction following parenteral methotrexate. There is no apparent gross intellectual impairment following successful treatment of leukemia prior to relapse. However, more detailed tests of children given prophylactic RT to the head together with systemic as well as intrathecal methotrexate are showing signs of defects. These include short-term memory problems and drops in IQ levels [18]. Long-term ovarian and testicular disorders – at least, gross hormonal dysfunctions – are not usually seen following treatment for leukemia unless gonadal irradiation has been included in the regimen. There are numerous reports now of successful childbearing after treatment for leukemia for 3–5 years.

The 1980s: Increase in Cure and Possible Prevention

During the last 4 decades, while clinicians were improving methods of treatment, laboratory researchers have been trying to understand the etiology of leukemia and the reasons for the disordered white cell growth. Differentiation sequences and membrane structure have been exhaustively examined. It is to be hoped that from studies such as these will come the means of eradicating the disease in all patients and possibly even preventing the leukemias. Prevention is one of the primary goals in pediatrics and prevention of such a devastating disease as leukemia would be the ultimate triumph.

References

1 Burchenal, J.H.; Ellison, R.R.; Murphy, M.L.; et al.: Clinical studies on 6-mercaptopurine. Ann. N. Y. Acad. Sci. *60:*359 (1954).
2 D'Angio, G.J.; Evans, A.E.; Mitus, A.: Roentgen therapy of certain complications of acute leukemia in childhood. Am. J. Roentg. *82:*541–553 (1959).
3 Dessauer, F.: Eine neue Anordnung zur Röntgenbestrahlung. Arch. phys. Med. med. Tech. *2:*218–223 (1905).
4 Farber, S.; Diamond, L.K.; Mercer, R.D.; et al.: Temporary remissions in acute leukemia in children produced by folic acid antagonist, *l*-amino-*p*-teroyl-glutamic acid (aminopterin). New Engl. J. Med. *238:*787–793 (1948).
5 Farber, S.; Schwathman, H.; Toch, R.; et al.: The effect of ACTH in acute leukemia in childhood; in Mote, Proc. First ACTH Conf., p. 328 (Blakiston, Philadelphia 1950).
6 Freireich, E.J.; Karon, M.; Frei, E. III: Quadruple combination therapy (VAMP) for acute lymphocytic leukemia of childhood. Proc. Am. Ass. Cancer Res. *5:* 20 (1964).
7 Freireich, E.J.; Karon, M.; Flatow, F.; Frei, E., III: Effect of intensive cyclic chemotherapy (BIKE) on remission duration in acute lymphocytic leukemia. Proc. Am. Ass. Cancer Res. *6:*20 (1965).
8 George, P.; Hernandez, K.; Hustu, O.; et al.: A study of 'total therapy' of acute lymphocytic leukemia in children. J. Pediat. *72:*399–408 (1968).
9 Hammond, G.D.: Progress in the study, treatment and cure of the cancers of children; in Burchenal, Oettgen, Cancer: achievements, challenges and prospects for the 1980s, pp. 171–190 (Grune & Stratton, New York 1981).
10 Hann, H.-W. L.; Lustbader, E.D.; Evans, A.E.; et al.: Lack of influence of T-cell marker and importance of mediastinal mass on the prognosis of acute lymphocytic leukemias of childhood. J. natn. Cancer Inst. *66:*285–290 (1981).
11 Henderson, E.S.: Combination chemotherapy of acute lymphocytic leukemia of childhood. Cancer Res. *27:*2570 (1967).
12 Heyn, R.M.; Joo, P.; Karon, M.; et al.: BCG in the treatment of acute lymphocytic leukemia. Blood *46:*431 (1975).
13 Jacobson, L.O.; Spurr, C.L.; Barron, E.S.G.; et al.: Nitrogen mustard therapy. J. Am. med. Ass. *132:*263–271 (1947).
14 Kim, T.; Nesbit, M.; D'Angio, G.J.; Levitt, S.H.: The role of CNS irradiation in children with acute lymphoblastic leukemia. Radiology *104:*635–641 (1972).
15 Krivit, W.; Brubaker, C.; Thatcher, L.B.; et al.: Maintenance therapy in acute leukemia of childhood. Comparison of cyclic vs. sequential methods. Cancer *21:* 352 (1968).

16 Mathé, G.; Schwarzenberg, L.; Mery, A..M.; et al.: Extensive histological and psychological survey of patients with acute leukemia in 'complete remission'. Br. med. J. *121*: 642 (1966).

17 Mathé, G.; Amiel, J.L.; Schwarzenberg, L.; et al.: Active immunotherapy for acute lymphoblastic leukemia. Lancet *i*: 697 (1969).

18 Meadows, A.T.; Gordon, J.; Littman, P.; et al.: Pattern of cognitive dysfunctions in children with acute lymphocytic leukemia (ALL) treated with cranial irradiation. Proc. Am. Soc. clin. Oncol. *21*: 386 (1980).

19 Medical Research Council: Treatment of acute lymphoblastic leukemia. Comparison of immunotherapy (BCG), intermittent methotrexate and no therapy after a 5-month intensive cytotoxic regimen. Concord trial. Br. med. J. *iv*: 189 (1971).

20 Miller, D.R.; Leikin, S.; Albo, V.; et al.: Intensive induction and maintenance therapy in acute lymphoblastic leukemia of childhood – CCG 141. The role of prognostic factors. Blood (in press).

21 Minot, G.R.; Buckman, T.E.; Isaacs, R.: Chronic myelogenous leukemia. Age incidence, duration and benefit derived from irradiation. J. Am. med. Ass. *82*: 1489–1494 (1924).

22 Ortega, J.A.; Nesbit, M.E.; Donaldson, M.H.; et al.: *L*'Asparaginase, vincristine and prednisone for induction of first remission in acute lymphocytic leukemia. Cancer Res. *37*: 535 (1977).

23 Pearson, O.H.; Eliel, L.P.; Talbot, T.R., Jr.: The use of ACTH and cortisone in neoplastic diseases. Bull. N.Y. Acad. Med. *26*: 235 (1950).

24 Sather, H.; Miller, D.; Nesbit, M.; et al.: Differences in male/female prognosis for children with acute lymphoblastic leukemia (ALL). Proc. Am. Soc. Clin. Oncology *21*: 442 (1980).

25 Skipper, H.E.; Schabel, F.M., Jr.; Wilcox, W.S.: Experimental evaluation of potential anticancer agents. XIII. On the criteria and kinetics associated with 'curability' of experimental leukemia. Cancer Chemother. Rep. *35*: 1 (1964).

26 Thomas, E.D.; Herman, E.C.; Greenbaugh, W.B.; et al.: Irradiation and marrow infusion in leukemia. Archs intern. Med. *107*: 829–845 (1961).

27 Thomas, E.D.; Buckner, D.C.; Clift, R.H.; et al.: Marrow transplantation for acute non-lymphoblastic leukemia in first remission. New Engl. J. Med. *301*: 597–599 (1979).

28 Weinstein, H.J.; Mayer, R.J.; Rosenthal, D.S.; et al.: Treatment of acute myelogenous leukemia in children and adults. New Engl. J. Med. *303*: 473–478 (1980).

29 Whiteside, J.A.; Philips, F.S.; Dargeon, H.W.; et al.: Intrathecal amethopterin in neurological manifestations of leukemia. Archs intern. Med. *101*: 279–285 (1958).

30 Zeulzer, W.W.: Implications of long-term survival in acute stem cell leukemia of childhood treated with composite cyclic therapy. Blood *24*: 477 (1964).

A.E. Evans, MD, Children's Hospital of Philadelphia, Cancer Center, Division of Oncology, University of Pennsylvania, Philadelphia, PA 19104 (USA)

Front. Radiat. Ther. Onc., vol. 16, pp. 30–39 (Karger, Basel 1982)

Management of Children with Wilms' Tumor: Defining the Risk-Benefit Ratio[1]

G. D'Angio[a], *A. Evans*[a], *N. Breslow*[b], *E. Baum*[c], *J. B. Beckwith*[d], *A. deLorimier*[e], *D. Fernbach*[f], *E. Hrabovsky*[g], *B. Jones*[g], *P. Kelalis*[h], *H. B. Othersen, Jr*[i], *M. Tefft*[j], *P. Thomas*[k]

[a] Children's Cancer Research Center, Philadelphia, Pa., USA; [b] University of Washington, Seattle, Wash., USA; [c] Children's Memorial Hospital, Chicago, Ill., USA; [d] Children's Orthopedic Hospital, Seattle, Wash., USA; [e] University of California, San Francisco, Calif., USA; [f] Baylor College of Medicine, Houston, Tex., USA; [g] West Virginia University, Morgantown, W.Va., USA; [h] Mayo Clinic, Rochester, Minn., USA; [i] Medical University Hospital, Charleston, S.C., USA; [j] Rhode Island Hospital, Brown University, Providence, R.I., USA; [k] Washington University, St. Louis, Mo., USA

The management of patients with cancer is relatively straight-forward. One balances the short- and long-term risks of a specific treatment or set of treatments against the likely benefits to be achieved for the particular type of cancer, its stage, and its other features that are known to have prognostic import. The problem, of course, is defining the risk – benefit ratio with precision.

These problems in assessment are most prominent in the management of children with malignant diseases because of the well-known potential for early and late adversities associated with therapy, especially when potent antimitotic treatments such as irradiation or chemotherapy are employed in the developing child.

The several steps in the progress made against the Wilms' tumor trace the evolution of modern pediatric oncology, and were taken by weighing the potential gains of therapy against its hazards at several crucial points during the last several decades.

First, there were high risks merely in operating on small children

[1] Supported in part by USPHS grant No. CA-11722 and CA-14489.

with large abdominal tumors, and removal was seldom attempted. The operative mortality at one of the leading pediatric institutions was in the 20–25% range during the early years of this century. The specialty of pediatric surgery developed, and pioneering surgeons made the attempts more often. The operative mortality remained high, but the overall survival rose from less than 10 to 30%. Then anesthesia techniques, and pre-, intra-, and postoperative care advanced. Surgical mortality dropped to 3%, and there was a complementary rise in the survival to 40%. Clearly, there now was a net gain when trained surgeons attempted excision of the Wilms' tumor.

The radiosensitivity of Wilms' tumor had become apparent by this time, and irradiation was added by many as a routine post operative measure[1]. This was perhaps the first example of coordinated, multimodal care in pediatric oncology. A rise to a 47% 2 year survival rate was attributed to the use of routine post operative radiation therapy, but severe growth disturbances secondary to flank irradiation began to be recorded by several observers[15,16]. Methods for mitigating these problems were devised, and high energy beams with their skin and bone-sparing properties became available, but scoliosis and muscle fibrosis could not be avoided entirely[8]. Second neoplasms appeared; some were benign and some malignant. As the hazards became better defined, observers began to ask whether a patient with a tumor confined to the kidney and that was totally excised really needed to be irradiated. The question seemed particularly pertinent in babies who not only suffered the most damage, but also appeared to have a better overall outlook, especially when the tumors were diagnosed at an early stage.

Meanwhile, effective chemotherapy against leukemia was discovered. This stimulated a search for similarly effective agents against solid tumors, and actinomycin-D (AMD) and vincristine (VCR) soon were identified [5]. The use of these toxic substances as adjuvants was first resisted by both radiation therapists and surgeons because of uncertain benefits, and because they appeared to interfere with the care and well-being of children in the post operative period. Indeed, severe toxicity and occasional deaths attributed to chemotherapy did little to encourage their wide-spread use. Effective yet tolerable regimens nonetheless were evolved, better over-all survival rates were achieved; and when risks were weighed against benefits, a net gain could again be demonstrated. 80% of children receiving chemotherapy as well as radi-

Table I. National Wilms' Tumor Study Grouping System

The patient's group is decided by the surgeon in the operating room, and is confirmed by the pathologist. If the histological diagnosis and grouping will take more than 48 h, the surgical grouping stands, the patient is registered and started on treatment.

Group I: Tumor limited to kidney and completely excised.

The surface of the renal capsule is intact. The tumor was not ruptured before or during removal. There is no residual tumor apparent beyond the margins of excision.

Group II: Tumor extends beyond the kidney but is completely excised.

There is local extension of the tumor, i.e., penetration beyond the pseudocapsule into the perirenal soft tissues, or peri-aortic lymph node involvement. The renal vessels outside the kidney substance are infiltrated or contain tumor thrombus. There is no residual tumor apparent beyond the margins of excision.

Group III: Residual nonhematogenous tumor confined to abdomen.

Any one or more of the following occur: (1) the tumor has been biopsied or ruptured before or during surgery; (2) there are implants on peritoneal surfaces; (3) there are involved lymph nodes beyond the abdominal peri-aortic chains; (4) the tumor is not completely removable because of local infiltration into vital structures.

Group IV: Hematogenous metastases.

Deposits beyond group III; e.g., lung, liver, bone and brain.

Group V: Bilateral renal involvement either initially or subsequently.

---

ation therapy postoperatively survived 2 years, and the chemotherapist became an intregal third member of the therapeutic team.

These several steps, which took over a half-century, led to what is the basic tenet of modern therapy, i.e., coordinated, multimodal management. These steps were taken largely by individual investigators and groups of investigators working in single institutions. The next major advance was the creation of the cooperative study group. Investigators in individual institutions banded together to pool their patient and scientific resources, and thus made possible large-scale studies that yielded statistically significant results within reasonable periods of time. The first trials confirmed the efficacy of AMD and VCR in the management of these patients, and one such study indicated that protracted treatment with AMD gave results that were superior to a single para-operative course. Even more patients were needed, however, to

address the refinements of therapy that now assumed greater importance as the risks and benefits of therapy were weighed for subsets of
Wilms' tumor patients. It was time to answer whether routine postoperative radiation therapy was needed for early stage lesions that were
totally excised. There remained the question as to whether VCR was
superior to AMD, and whether the use of both agents would prove better still. Large numbers of patients were needed to answer these questions. The cooperative groups concerned with the study of childhood
cancer consolidated their Wilms' tumor inquiries and formed the
National Wilms' Tumor Study (NWTS) group. Patients were stratified
according to the extent of disease (table I), and were entered in randomized therapeutic trials. The NWTS group defined several other
research objectives. Epidemiologic information was to be accumulated, as were details regarding pathology, surgery, radiation therapy
and chemotherapy so that the appropriate analyses of these important
factors could be made.

The NWTS has shown that patients with group I tumors who are
given AMD and VCR postoperatively [4] enjoy excellent survival experience even though they are not irradiated (table II). Further, survival
rates are not significantly statistically different if AMD and VCR are
given such children for 6 months rather than for 15 months. A concrete
result is that the 230 group I children entered in NWTS-2 have been
spared the late consequences of flank irradiation without jeopardizing
their chances for relapse-free survival which, indeed, appears to have
improved. NWTS-1 also showed that for group II and III patients, all
of whom were irradiated, AMD plus VCR is superior to either agent
alone. In NWTS-2, better 2-year relapse-free survival rates for groups
II, III and IV were obtained when adriamycin (ADR) was added to the
other two agents (table II).

The exemplary cooperation of the hundreds of NWTS investigators has made other gains possible. The epidemiologic data collected
permitted NCI investigators to make more accurate estimates of the
frequency of congenital anomalies and to report certain familial
aspects of Wilms' tumor populations. Detailed cytohistopathologic
evaluations of thousands of specimens by Drs. *Beckwith, Palmer* and
their colleagues of the NWTS Pathology Center have led to the identification of microscopic features associated with specific patterns of disease evolution [3]. Survival rates of 89 and 39% at 2 years have been
recorded for histologic types grouped under the rubrics, 'favorable his-

Table II. Results of National Wilms' Tumor Study: Outcome by randomized groups and regimens

Group and regimen[1]	n	% 4-year relapse-free survival		% 4-year survival	
NWTS-1					
I < 2 years old					
A (RT)	38	89		94	
B (no RT)	41	88	p = 0.85	90	p = 0.46
I ≧ 2 years old					
A (RT)	42	76		98	
B (no RT)	42	57	p = 0.06	81	p = 0.015
II/III					
A (AMD)	63	56		71	
B (VCR)	44	57	p = 0.01	71	p = 0.01
C (AMD + VCR)	63	79		84	

	n	% 3-year relapse-free survival		% 3-year survival	
NWTS-2					
I					
E (short)	106	96		97	
F (long)	109	90	p = 0.21	91	p = 0.15
II/III/IV					
C	159	65		74	
D (+ADR)	155	79	p = 0,0006	84	p = 0.06

[1] Regimen   IA = Postoperative actinomycin D (AMD) for 15 months plus irradiation (RT)

            IB = Postoperative AMD for 15 months without RT

            IE = Postoperative AMD + vincristine (VCR) for 6 months without RT

            IF = Postoperative AMD + VCR for 15 months without RT

II/III/(IV)   A = Postoperative RT + AMD for 15 months

            B = Postoperative RT + VCR for 15 months

            C = Postoperative RT + AMD + VCR for 15 months

            D = Postoperative RT + AMD + VCR + adriamycin for 15 months.

See *D'Angio* et al. [3, 4] for additional details.

tology' (FH) and 'unfavorable histology' (UH), respectively. Included in the latter category are at least four subtypes: those with focal or with diffuse anaplasia, and those with sarcomatous features which have been termed the 'rhabdoid' and the 'clear cell' types. Indeed, the latter two neoplasms may not be Wilms' tumor at all; at least, the 'rhabdoid' has been identified in extrarenal structures. It is of considerable interest that the rhabdoid tumor tends to be associated with cerebral lesions. These take either of two forms: metastases or independent brain tumors of small cell type. The clear cell sarcoma, on the other hand, has a propensity to metastasize to bone, and has been described independently by *Marsden* et al. [12] as 'bone-metastasizing renal tumor of childhood'. These observations have obvious connotations insofar as what type of roentgen and other diagnostic studies should be performed at the time of diagnosis and thereafter [3].

Statistical analyses of the gross and microscopic features of Wilms' tumor have identified various other factors which are of prognostic importance. Most prominent among these after histologic type is the presence of lymph node metastases, a finding that confirms earlier observations reported by *Jereb and Eklund* [9]. Details relevant to surgical technique were evaluated with several interesting results. For example, biopsies and minor nicks of the tumor capsule at the time of surgery were not associated with an unfavorable outcome. Radiation therapy factors were also analyzed and no distinct dose-response relationships emerged from retrospective analyses of pooled data. No special advantage could be detected in patients who received postoperative irradiation within a day or two of surgery (as was thought by some to be important); on the other hand, results suggested that delays of 10 or more days were associated with less favorable survival.

These and other observations led to a modification of the grouping method that was employed in the first two studies. NWTS-3 uses a new staging system that promises to be better. This expectation was tested by comparing the survival rates of randomized NWTS-2 patients according to the group originally assigned and after the same patients were retrospectively reassigned according to the new staging criteria[6]. Projected survival for stage I, II and III children was rank-ordered more clearly than when the grouping system was employed. This latter exercise demonstrates another use that can be made of data filed in cooperative studies; that is, the accumulated material can be used to test hypotheses or for other ancillary studies [7].

Refinements of Wilms' tumor therapy are still sought in order to define the risk-benefit ratios with greater precision for smaller and smaller subsets of children. Appropriate cooperative group research is underway by investigators in the United Kingdom and those participating in the studies of the International Society of Pediatric Oncology (SIOP). Both groups have made noteworthy contributions. The British team has shown that more intensive and sustained VCR therapy gives superior results. SIOP demonstrated that preoperative irradiation lessened the risk of tumor rupture [10, 14]. NWTS-3 also is designed to refine therapy, as were NWTS-1 and NWTS-2. An important research concept that is receiving increasing emphasis and is part of NWTS-3, is the search for reductions in therapy that will nonetheless yield good results. This is especially important in children, of course, but also is dictated by the successes of pediatric oncology. Reductions of treatment in pursuit of lower and lower risk-benefit ratios is at least as important as increasing therapy in the chase for better and better survival rates. It is practically impossible to improve the excellent survival for early stage, FH tumors with current therapy, for example. Thus, in NWTS-3, reduced chemotherapy and radiation therapy is being tested for group I FH patients who are at relatively low risk from their disease (fig. 1). Those at high risk are not neglected, of course, and better survival is being sought for group IV children and all those with UH tumors by increasing the intensity of therapy (fig. 1). Doubts regarding the risk-benefit ratios of certain current therapies remain, and these will be resolved in part by longitudinal studies of long-term survivors. The potential for late adversities is enhanced after combined modality care because of irradiation-drug interactions as well as the effects of each agent itself. Late cardiac damage associated with ADR given young children, even though it appears to be tolerated in the short term, is one such doubt. For this reason, NWTS-3 seeks to determine whether a more intense course of AMD and VCR will give results equal to those achieved with AMD, VCR and ADR.

It is obvious that definition of the risk-benefit ratio remains a principal objective of those who manage children with Wilms' tumor. Only by more precise understanding of the benefits and hazards of treatment vis-à-vis stage, age, tumor type, and the myriad of other factors that make up the Wilms' tumor complex can the therapist be sure he is doing the best for his patient not only for today but also for tomorrow and the day after.

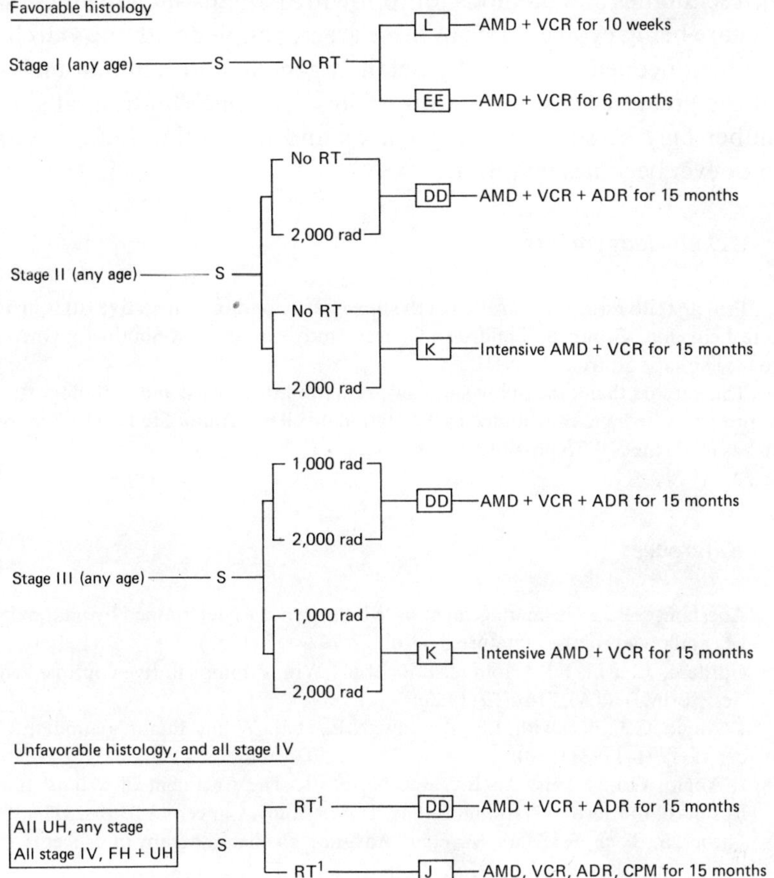

Fig. 1. National Wilms' Tumor Study-3. FH = Favorable histology; UH = unfavorable histology; RT = irradiation; S = surgery; L, EE, DD, K and J = chemotherapy regimens indicated on the schema.
[1] All FH stage IV receive 2,000 rad flank RT and RT to other sites as in NWTS-2. All UH, all stages, receive age-adjusted flank RT and to other sites as in NWTS-2.

Meanwhile, studies by other investigators are identifying with greater precision the patient or the family at high risk for developing Wilms' tumor. The well-known associations of the neoplasm with aniridia, hemi-hypertrophy, the Beckwith-Wiedemann syndrome, or the presence of nephroblastomatosis all put the patients with these pathologies at high risk for the eventual appearance of Wilms' tumor [2, 11,

13]. Techniques and methods for following patients showing these stigmata are being evolved. It is in these areas, coupled with the search for possible oncogens [17] and by detailed genetic and familial analyses, that the greatest hope for the future lies for some children, albeit the number may be small: in prophylaxis and prevention before Wilms' tumor ever becomes manifest.

Acknowledgements

Principal investigators enrolled in the three participating cooperative study groups, Acute Leukemia Group B, Children's Cancer Study Group, and Southwest Oncology also receive support from the NIH.

The authors thank the many surgeons, radiation therapists, and pathologists, past and present, who have contributed to the National Wilms' Tumor Study. Their cooperation has made the NWTS possible.

References

1   Abeshouse, B.J.: The management of Wilms' tumor as determined by national survey and review of the literature. J. Urol. *77:*792–813 (1957).
2   Cordero, J.F.; Li, F.P.; Holmes, L.B., et al.: Wilms' tumor in five cousins. Pediatrics, Springfield *66:*716–719 (1980).
3   D'Angio, G.J.; Beckwith, J.B.; Breslow, N.E., et al.: Wilms' tumor: an update. Cancer *45:*1791–1798 (1980).
4   D'Angio, G.J.; Evans, A.; Breslow, N., et al.: The treatment of Wilms' tumor. Results of the Second National Wilms' Tumor Study. Cancer *47:*2302–2311 (1981).
5   Farber, S.; Toch, R.; Sears, M., et al.: Advances in chemotherapy of cancer in man. Adv. Cancer Res. *4:*1–71 (1956).
6   Farewell, V.T.; D'Angio, G.J.; Breslow, N.; Norkool, P.: Retrospective validation of a new staging system for Wilms' tumor. A report from the National Wilms' Tumor Study. Cancer clin. Trials *4:*167–171 (1981).
7   Farewell, V.T.; D'Angio, G.J.: A simulated study of historical controls using real data. Biometrics *37:*169–176 (1981).
8   Heaston, D.K.; Libshitz, H.I.; Chan, R.C.: Skeletal effects of megavoltage irradiation in survivors of Wilms' tumor. Am. J. Roentg. *133:*389–395 (1979).
9   Jereb, B.; Eklund, G.: Factors influencing the cure rate in nephroblastoma. Acta radiol. *12:*84–106 (1973).
10 Lemerle, J.; Voute, P.A.; Tournade, M.F., et al.: Preoperative versus postoperative radiotherapy, single versus multiple course of actinomycin D, in the treatment of Wilms' tumor. Cancer *38:*647–654 (1976).
11 Machin, G.A.: Persistent renal blastema (nephroblastomatosis) as a frequent precursor of Wilms' tumor; a pathological and clinical review. III. Clinical aspects of nephroblastomatosis. Am. J. Ped. Hematol./Oncol. *2:*353–362 (1980).

12   Marsden, H.B.; Lawler, W.; Kumar, P.M.: Bone metastasizing renal tumor of child-
     hood. Morphological and clinical features, and differences from Wilms' tumor.
     Cancer 42:1922–1928 (1978).
13   Miller, R.W.: Cancer and congenital malformations: another view; in Mulvihill,
     Miller, Fraumeni, Genetics in human cancer, pp. 77–81 (Raven press, New York,
     1977).
14   Morris-Jones, P.H.: Medical Research Council's Working Party on Embryonal
     Tumors in Childhood. Management of nephroblastoma in childhood. Archs. Dis.
     Childh. 53:112–119 (1978).
15   Rubin, P.; Duthie, R.B.; Young, L.W.: The significance of scoliosis in post-irradi-
     ated Wilms' tumor and neuroblastoma. Radiology 79:539–559 (1962).
16   Vaeth, J.M.; Levitt, S.W.; Jones, M.D.; Holtfreter, C.: Effects of radiation therapy
     in survivours of Wilms' tumor. Radiology 79:560–568 (1962).
17   Zack, M.; Cannon, S.; Loyd, D.; Heath, C., Jr.; Falletta, J.; Jones, B.; Housworth,
     J.; Crowley, S.: Cancer in children of parents exposed to hydrocarbon related
     industries and occupations. Epidemiology 3:329–336 (1980).

G.J. D'Angio, MD, Director, Children's Cancer Research Center,
Children's Hospital of Philadelphia, Philadelphia, PA 19104 (USA)

Front. Radiat. Ther. Onc., vol. 16, pp. 40–41 (Karger, Basel 1982)

Discussion

Feusner: What is the advantage of pre- or intraoperative chemotherapy or radiotherapy for Wilms's tumor?

D'Angio: I do not think that we have any evidence suggesting that preoperative or intraoperative chemotherapy or radiation therapy confers a survival advantage. In the first SIPO study (International Society of Pediatric Oncology), patients were randomized to receive preoperative irradiation or postoperative radiation therapy. The survival was the same in the two groups. Those patients who were irradiated preoperatively hat fewer intraoperative ruptures of tumor, however. The SIPO study cogently suggests that in girls this seems to make a big difference, since it is not necessary to give total abdominal and, thus, overian irradiation to the patients who do not rupture. I do not think that there is any evidence suggesting that preoperative chemotherapy confers a survival advantage, i.e., at least according to our own and accumulated data. SIPO is currently concerned with this question, so as far as I am concerned, there is no major advantage, except the one I have already indicated. It makes surgery easier. On occasion, we certainly do perform preoperative irradiation even at the Children's Hospital in Philadelphia. When an experienced surgeon has detected a tumor which is so massive that he fears the morbidity and possible mortality, we do oblige by giving preoperative therapy. As a routine though, I do not think it has much of an advantage; if anything, then a disadvantage, namely, that one cannot always differentiate entirely benign tumors, like polycystic kidneys, no matter how carefully the preoperative evaluation is done. Inappropriate therapy could be given to a proportion of these patients constituting about 8% of the sample.

Audience: Dr. *Austin,* much has not been said about etiologies in childhood leukemia or cancer in general. You did not mention specifically agents that may cross the placenta and affect the newborn. I wonder if you would care to comment on that.

Austin: I did not mention such agents specifically, because I was not very sure about which ones were valid and which ones were not. I do not have a very good understanding of which ones are likely to be etiologic agents.

Audience: What is your opinion about the effects of diethylstilbesterol and perhaps even of Dilantin in childhood?

Austin: Diethylstilbesterol is not carcinogenic in the sense of initiating malignant cells itself, but, rather, it causes an abnormality in the development of the fetus such that there are susceptible cells left which normally would not be there. It causes the development of an entire clone of abnormal cells which is very susceptible to carcinogenesis. None of the hormones, as a matter of fact, shows carcinogenic effects or mutogenic effects when tested in bacterial systems. Dilantin has the possibility of being a carcinogen which may cross the placental barrier, as a number of other agents which we really do not have enough information about right now.

Audience: Regarding Dilantin there are a couple of curious reports on neuroblastomas occurring in the offspring of mothers receiving this agent.

Audience: Dr. *Evans,* I would like to congratulate you on a very elucidating talk. I have not heard many like yours outlining the progression of leukemia therapy over the years.

You made many comments on prognostic factors for ALL, and I wonder if you would like to make some comments on prognostic factors for AML, the nonlymphocytic group?

Evans: I do not know a great deal about the prognostic factors for AML, in part because I do not think they have been studied enough, and also, if you have poor survival on the whole, you are not able to separate the patients' 'bad' symptoms. One of the problems we have in AML is a drop-off rate early in diagnosis. It is a disease with early hemorrhage. There is a significant drop-off in number of patients right at the beginning. I have not undertaken any particular studies on prognosis in AML.

Dr. *Austin,* I would like to go back to one of your comments, and I may have misunderstood one of your slides. It seemed to me that you showed a slide which showed the best survival or prognosis in acute leukemia to be in the first 4 years of life, and it may be that the majority of children in that age-group were 2 or 3 years old which improved the survival. We would put the best prognosis in a slightly older age-group.

Austin: You are probably right in explaining why the 0–1 age-group did not show up. We lumped together 0 through 4 years, and it is also quite true that children diagnosed during the first year of life constitute a very small percentage of the number diagnosed in the first 5 years of life.

Van Eys: I would like to make a footnote to Dr. *Evans* talk. The pediatric oncology group just reviewed all of our leukemia data, and we worked on prognostic factors one step beyond these data to see if they may, in fact, be representative of a hidden disease. The later data were extremely interesting revealing that there are specific leukemias that have been lumped together as ALL which are not only unique by grouping prognostic factors but, in fact, biologically, clinically, immunologically, and morphologically. The newest addition to this group is the pre-B-cell leukemia, which is characterized by cytoplasmic immunoglobulins with B cell behavior ability of immunologic characteristics. These patients do as poorly as T cell leukemia patients, although by prognostic factors at initial diagnosis they are not distinguishable from pre-B-cell leukemia. I think that we are now at the next step where we should not talk about stage, anymore, but we should, in fact, accept the fact that lymphocytic leukemia can be subdivided in to at least six different diseases that are biologically unique. I wonder if Dr. *Evans* would comment on the CCFG efforts in the same direction.

Evans: I agree with you that we should consider the biology of leukemia and not simply numbers. I think many of our prognostic associations are simply the biology of a disease which may have different courses and may be entirely different diseases. If you look at the bone marrow of a child with a lymphoma syndrome and another child with acute leukemia, you would not be able to tell the difference by looking at the cells, but other symptoms would tell you that they may be two entirely different diseases. I know that we have too few children with B cell leukemia with a bad prognosis to be able to distinguish it as a disease; although, if you have a child with B cell leukemia, you know it is a difficult case. Concerning the T cell markers, it is interesting to show that if you look at the other data and the height of the white count and so forth, the effect of T cells is not very strong. It is a bad prognostic factor, since it is associated with a very high white count very often and sometimes with a mediastinal mass; the white count is the stronger variable. T cell disease alone is not bad. Dr. Hahn reports that a girl without a high white count and a mediastinal mass or other disease, suffering from T cell disease has a very good prognosis; this shows that the T cell alone is not enough.

Front. Radiat. Ther. Onc., vol. 16, pp. 42–49 (Karger, Basel 1982)

The Relative Tolerance of Children and Adults to Anticancer Drugs

Daniel L. Glaubiger[a], *Daniel D. von Hoff*[b], *John S. Holcenberg*[c], *Bart Kamen*[c], *Charles Pratt*[d], *Richard S. Ungerleider*[e]

[a] Pediatric Oncology Branch, Clinical Oncology Program, Division of Cancer Treatment, National Cancer Institute, Bethesda, Md., USA; [b] Division of Oncology, Department of Medicine, University of Texas at San Antonio, Tex., USA; [c] Milwaukee Children's Hospital, Medical College of Wisconsin, Milwaukee, Wisc., USA; [d] St. Jude's Children's Research Hospital; [e] Clinical Investigations Branch, Cancer Therapy Evaluation Program, Division of Cancer Treatment, National Cancer Institute, Bethesda, Md., USA

Patients with childhood malignancies represent a small fraction of the total cancer patient population and the malignancies that do occur in children are relatively uncommon. Nonetheless, the neoplasms that are more common in younger patients have proved to be far more tractable to therapy than adult tumors and, in fact, the majority of active anticancer drugs are effective against childhood tumors.

While the spectrum of antitumor activity, for many agents, differs between adults and children, the toxicities associated with the administration of these agents have been thought to be similar in both age groups. On that basis, as well as the relatively low frequency of childhood cancer, it has been thought that toxicity trials of new anticancer agents specifically directed at the pediatric patient population were not necessary. I order to examine this question more fully, we have reviewed that data available on those anticancer drugs which have had formal, comparable, toxicity trials in both adult and pediatric patients. We have compared the spectrum of toxic effects observed in both patient groups as well as the relative tolerance of patients for these drugs, as reflected by the maximally tolerated doses defined in the trials.

Approximately 90 antitumor drugs have had formal toxicity trials in patients with cancer as part of the screening program of the

Table I. Drugs with phase I trials in children

Drug	NSC number
Adriamycin	123127
5-Azacytidine	102816
Azaserine	742
Cyclocytidine	145668
Anhydro-5-fluoro-cyclocytidine	166641
Daunomycin	82151
Dianhydrogalactitol	132313
Diglycoaldehyde	118994
Piperazinedione	135758
TIC mustard	82196
VM-26	122819
VP16-213	141540
β-TGdR	71261
2'-Deoxycoformycin	218321
3-Deazauridine	126849
m-Amsa	141549
Dihydroxyanthracenedione	301739
ICRF-187	169780

National Cancer Institute . Of these 90 drugs, 20 have had toxicity trials directed at pediatric patients. These 2 compounds are listed in table I. Although the precise biochemical mechanisms of antitumor activity are not known for all these drugs, they come from several distinct classes of active agents, in terms of their mechanisms of cytotoxicity. They include alkylating agents, such as TIC Mustard (NSC 82196), intercalating agents like adriamycin (NSC 123127) and m-Amsa (NSC 141549), antimetabolites such as 2'-deoxycoformycin and 5-azacytidine (NSC 102816), and tubulin antagonists such as VM-26 (NSC 122819) and VP16-213 (NSC 141540). Overall similarities in toxic effects seen in both patient groups could not, therefore, be ascribed to similarities among the drugs tested, with regard to the mechanism of action.

Toxic effects observed in trials of these compounds in pediatric and adult patient populations were similar, in terms of the organ systems affected. In some cases, however, differences in toxicity were noted. Skin rashes were seen in children given daunomycin (NSC 82151) or adriamycin (NSC 123127), but not in adult patients given the same drugs [1, 16]. Fever was noted in adult patients given azaserine (NSC 742) but not in children [3].

In some instances, more significant differences have been observed. The hydrazine derivatives procarbazine (NSC 77213) and azapicyl (NSC 68626) have not had directly comparable trials in adults and children. However, marked differences in toxicity were noted during clinical trials of the two compounds, with seizures and neuropathies being seen in adult patients but not in children [6, 8, 14, 15]. In general, the severity of the toxicities common to both groups of patients tends to be higher in adults. This has been noted for some time with drugs such as vincristine (NSC 67574) where neurologic side effects including arthralgias, myalgias and ileus have been noted to be more frequent and to occur at lower dose levels in adults than in children [11, 12]. It is particularly true for the drug 2'-deoxycoformycin (NSC 218321), an analog of adenine which inhibits the enzyme adenosine deaminase, and has only recently completed toxicity trials in pediatric patients [10]. Severe renal and neuromuscular toxicities were noted in adult patients receiving the drug, necessitating discontinuance of toxicity trials of the drug in this patient group. Significant toxic effects were noted in children only at much higher drug doses, approximately three times the maximum dosage given to adults before the trial was terminated.

If we now focus attention on those drugs which have had toxicity trials on the same schedule in both adults and children (e. g. daily 5×, every 3 weeks, etc.), and for which maximally tolerated doses have been determined in both patient groups, it is clear that the dose-limiting toxicity (that toxic effect of the drug which prevents further escalation of the dose on the schedule being tested) is the same for both adults and children. There are 16 compounds which have had clinical toxicity trials that meet the criteria outlined above. Table II shows a list of these drugs, the schedule which was tested in both adult and pediatric patient groups, and the dose-limiting toxicity observed in each group. Results for the compound ICRF-187, which is the d^+-enantiomer of ICRF-159, a previosly tested drug, are not shown because the toxicity trials in pediatric patients are not yet complete. (The trials have not defined a maximally tolerated dose for patients with solid tumors or for patients with leukemia.) The dose-limiting toxicity in adults with solid tumors is myelosuppression [5]. Of the 15 compounds for which comparable toxicity trials have been completed, all but one have the

Tabelle II. Comparison of dose-limiting toxicities (DTL) of anti cancer agents in children and adults

Drug	Schedule	DLT in Children	DLT in Adults
Dianhydrogalactitol	q.d.X5	myelosuppression	myelosuppression
5-Azacytidine	q.d. X5	myelosuppression	myelosuppression
TIC mustard	q.d. X5	gastrointestinal	gastrointestinal
Piperazinedione	q.d. X5	myelosuppression	myelosuppression
Diglycoaldehyde	q.d. X5	renal tubular damage	renal tubular damage
Daunomycin	q.d. X4	myelosuppression	myelosuppression
Adriamycin	q.d. X4	myelosuppressin	myelosuppression
VM-26	biweekly	myelosuppression	myelosuppression
VP16-213	biweekly	myelosuppression	myelosuppression
Azaserine	q.d.	mucositis	mucositis
Cyclocytidine	q.d. X10	myelosuppression	myelosuppression, hypotension
Anhydro-5-fluoro-cyclocytidine	q.d.	myelosuppression	myelosuppression
3-Deazauridine (leukemia patients)	q.d. X5	stomatitis	stomatitis
3-Deazauridine (solid tumor patients)	Q.D. X5	myelosuppression	myelosuppression
m-AMSA (solid tumor patients)	q.d. X5	myelosuppression	myelosuppression
m-AMSA (leukemia patients)	q.d. X5	stomatitis	stomatitis
Dihydroxyanthracene-dione	every 3 weeks	myelosuppression	myelosuppression

same dose-limiting toxicity in children and adults. Cyclocytidine (NSC 145668) was observed to have drug-associated hypotension as a dose-limiting toxic effect in adults but not in children [4, 7]. Myelosuppression was also dose-limiting in adult patients receiving cyclocytidine, and was the dose-limiting toxicity in pediatric patients. In fact, as can be seen in table II, myelosuppression was the dose-limiting toxicity for 13 of the 15 agents which have had comparable trials in both patient groups.

The comparison of maximally tolerated doses, determined for adults and children in formal clinical toxicity trials of antineoplastic agents, is shown in table III. Results are shown for drugs which have had trials on the same schedule in both patient groups. Some older tri-

Table III. Comparison of maximally tolerated doses (MTD) of anticancer agents in children and adults

Drug	Schedule	MTD mg/m²		Ratio MTD children: MTD adults
		children,	adults	
Dianhydrogalactitiol	q.d. X5	25	30	0.83
5-azacytidine	q.d. X5	200	225	0.89
TIC Mustard	q.d. X5	900	1,000	0.90
Piperazinedione	q.d. X5	3	3	1.0
VP16-213	biweekly	150	125	1.20
Diglycoaldehyde	q.d. X5	7,500⁺	6,000	1,25
m-AMSA	q.d. X5	50	40	1.25
Daunomycin mg/kg	q.d. X4	1.0	0.8	1.25
Adriamycin, mg/kg	q.d. X4	0.8	0.6	1.33
VM-26, mg/kg	biweekly	4.0	3.0	1.33
3-Deazauridine (leukemia patients)	q.d. X5	8.2	6.0	1.40
Azaserine, mg/kg (total dose)	q.d.	156	108	1.44
Anhydro-5-fluoro-cyclocyti-dine	q.d.	300⁺	200⁺	1.50
Dihydroxyanthracenedione	every 3 weeks	18	12	1.5
3-Deazauridine (solid tumors)	q.d. X5	2.8	1.5	1.85
Cyclocytidine	q.d. X10	600	300	2.00
ICRF-187	q.d. X3	>2,750	1,250	>2.20

als are included, in which doses were given on a milligrams per kilogram basis rather than a milligrams per square meter surface area basis. The overall data shown in table III indicate that, for 12 of the 16 drugs that have had comparable trials, the maximally tolerated dose defined for children is higher than that determined for adults. For one drug, piperazinedione (NSC 135758), maximally tolerated doses are equal for both groups, and, for three drugs, TIC mustard (NSC 82196), 5-azacytidine (NSC 102816), and dianhydrogalactitol (NSC 132313), pediatric patients tolerated less drug than adults, with the minimum ratio of tolerated doses being approximately five sixths (0.83). For those agents which were better tolerated by pediatric patients, the ratio of maximally tolerated doses (children/adults) was as high as 2.5 for ICRF-187.

Table IV. Therapeutic dosages of methotrexate in humans

	Infants	Older child	Adult
Weight, kg	8.0	20.0	70.0
Surface area m²	0.4	0.8	1.85
Daily dose, mg/kg	0.15	0.12	0.07
Daily dose mg/m²	3.1	3.1	2.7

The origins of the improved tolerance of pediatric patients for anticancer drugs is not certain. One possible explanation may lie in age-related differences in drug metabolism and excretion. There is some data obtained with the drug cyclophosphamide (NSC 26271) which supports this view [13]. Also, as has been pointed out using the drug methotrexate as an example, pediatric patients generally tolerate more drug on a milligrams per kilogram basis than adults, but tolerate similar drug doses based upon surface area [9]. A comparison of the relative doses is shown in table IV. As shown, the bulk of the difference in drug dose between adults and children (on a milligrams per kilogram basis) disappears when dosages are computed in terms of milligrams per square meter surface area. There remains, however, about a 10% difference in tolerable drug doses in favor of pediatric patients that is not accounted for, implying that, even after comparing drug doses in terms of surface area, children may have an excess metabolic or excretory rate for these drugs compared with adults. Differences in intracellular metabolic rates that were age dependent could also help to account for the observed differences.

Another possible explanation may lie in the fact that the majority of drugs tested had myelosuppression as the dose-limiting toxicity in both patient groups. A plausible hypothesis for the increased drug tolerance of children would be that they have larger numbers of hematopoietic stem cells per unit surface area compared with older patients. This is attractive, since the drugs evaluated come from different classes of compounds, in terms of molecular structure and mechanism of action, and would therfore not be expected to share common metabolic or excretory patterns. They do, however, have as a common effect, cytotoxicity for hematopoietic stem cells. There is, at present, no data which measures relative numbers of bone marrow stem cells as a function of age. However, the experience that is available indicates that the number of pluripotent bone marrow stem cells may diminish with advancing age [2].

Irrespective of possible explanations, it is clear that pediatric patients generally tolerate higher doses of anticancer drugs than do adults. If the evaluation of the antitumor activity of new drugs necessitates their being used at maximally tolerated doses, which has been one of the basic tenets of drug screening, then the data presented here suggest that maximally tolerated doses defined in adult toxicity trials are not valid for pediatric patients, and that children usually require higher drug doses to achieve optimum antitumor effects. This appears to be true for a number of drugs which are structurally unrelated and come from several different classes of agents, in terms of biochemical mechanism of action. The excess tolerance of pediatric patients for antineoplastic agents is variable, and, at present, not predictable. These results therefore indicate that toxicity trials specifically directed toward the pediatric age group are needed as part of the initial clinical assessment of new agents, in order to derive doses which are appropriate for subsequent evaluation of the antitumor activity of these agents in childhood cancer. They also indicate that such pediatric trials could be started at approximatels 80% of the maximally tolerated dose determined in adult trials and escalated from that point.

References

1   Bonadonna, G.; Monfardini, S.; Guindani, A.: Daunomycin treatment in chronic lymphoproliferative disorders. Tumori *54:* 465 (1968).
2   Bull, J.M.; Rubin, P.C.: Personal communication (1981).
3   Ellison, R.R.; Karnofsky, D.A.; Sternberg, S.S.; Murphy, M.L.; Burchenal, J.H.: Clinical trials of *o*-diazoacetyl-*L*-serine (azaserine) in neoplastic disease. Cancer *7:* 801 (1954).
4   Finkelstein, J.Z.; Higgins, G.; Krivit, W.; Hamond, D.: Evaluation of cyclocytidine in advanced leukemia and solid tumors. Cancer Treat. Rep. *63:* 1331 (1979).
5   Howser, D.; Lewis, B.J.; Young, R.C.; Weiss, R.B.; Hoff, D.D. von: Phase I trial of ICRF-187 (NSC 169780). Proc. Am. Ass. Cancer Res. *21:* 172 (1980).
6   Livingston, R.B.; Carter, S.K.: Procarbazine; in Single agents in cancer chemotherapy, pp. 318–336 (Plenum Press, New York 1970).
7   Lokich, J.J.; Chawla, P.L.; Jaffe, N.; Frei, E., III: Phase I evaluation of cyclocytidine (NSC 145668). Cancer Chemother. Rep. *59:* 389 (1975).
8   Olson, K.B.; Horton, J.; Pratt, K.L.; Paladine, W.J., Jr.; Cunningham, T.; Sullivan, J.; Hosley, H.; Treble, D.H.: 1-acetyl-2-picolinoylhydrazine (NSC 68626) in the treatment of advanced cancer. Cancer Chemother. Rep. *53:* 291 (1969).

9 Pinkel, D.: The use of body surface area as a criterion of drug dosage in cancer chemotherapy. Cancer Res. *18:*853 (1958).

10 Poplack, D.G.; Sallan, S.E..; Rivera, G.; Holcenberg, J.; Murphy, S.B.; Blatt, J.; Lipton, J.M.; Venner, P.; Glaubiger, D.L.; Ungerleider, R.S.; Johns, D.G.: Phase I study of 2'-deoxycoformycin in acute lymphoblastic leukemia. Cancer Res. (in press).

11 Sandler, S.G.; Tobin, W.; Henderson, E.S.: Vincristine induced neuropathy: a clinical study of fifty leukemic patients. Neurology, Minneap. *19:*367 (1969).

12 Selawry, O.S.; Hananian, J.: Vincristine treatment of cancer in children. J. Am. med. Ass. *183:*741 (1963).

13 Sladek, N.E.; Priest, J.; Doeden, J.; Mirocha, C.J.; Pathre, S.; Krivit, W.: Plasma half-life and urinary excretion of cyclophosphamide in children. Cancer Treat. Rep. *64:*1061 (1980).

14 Sutow, W.W.; Komp, D.; Vietti, T.J.; Pinkerton, D.: Clinical trials with 1-acetyl 2-picolinoylhydrazine (NSC 68626) in children. Cancer Chemother. Rep. *59:*341 (1975).

15 Stolinsky, D.C.; Solomon, J.; Pugh, R.P.; Stevens, A.R.; Jacobs, E.M.; Irvin, L.E.; Wood, D.A.: Clinical experience with procarbazine in Hodgkin's disease, reticulum cell sarcoma, and lymphosarcoma. Cancer *26:*984 (1970).

14 Tan, C.; Tasaka, H.; Kuo-Ping, Y.; Murphy, M.L.; Karnofsky, D.A.: Daunomycin, an antitumor antibiotic in the treatment of neoplastic disease : clinical evaluation with special reference to childhood leukemia. Cancer *20:*333 (1967).

D.L. Glaubiger, MD, Pediatric Oncology Branch, Clinical Oncology Program, Division of Cancer Treatment, National Cancer Institute, Bethesda, MD 20205 (USA)

Front. Radiat. Ther. Onc., vol. 16, pp. 50–54 (Karger, Basel 1982)

Delayed Toxicities of Chemotherapy on Childhood Tissues
1981 Update

W. Archie Bleyer[1]

Children's Orthopedic Hospital and Medical Center, University of Washington,
Fred Hutchinson Cancer Research Center, Seattle, Wash., USA

The *acute* adverse effects of cancer chemotherapy are tolerated better by children than by adults, as documented quantitatively in the report by *Glaubiger* et al. [this volume]. Conversely, however, the young child may be more vulnerable to the *delayed* sequelae of cancer chemotherapy. In this report I will review the current studies which address this issue, with particular reference to critical target tissues in the growing child.

Brain

In a cohort of 110 5-year survivors of childhood leukemia, the Late Effects Study Group (LESG) observed that 21 (19%) had significant sequelae [8]. The most frequently occurring residua were those related to the CNS, with 8 patients reported affected. Learning disability was noted in 5, encephalopathy in 2, and a seizure disorder in 1 patient. All of these children had received cranial radiation (Cr RT) 2,400 rad and intrathecal methotrexate (IT MTX) for prevention of CNS leukemia. Although 57% of the children were less than 5 years of age at diagnosis, 7 of the 8 patients with brain sequelae ware in that age group. A minimum of 11% of the children diagnosed before the age of 5 were estimated to have obvious deficits of intellectual function presumed secondary to therapy [8].

IQ testing in children regarded cured of acute lymphocytic leukemia (ALL) has revealed consistent findings in several recent studies, whether retrospective [4, 9] or prospective [7], controlled [7, 9] or uncontrolled [4]: (1) long-term survivors of childhood ALL treated with

---

[1] Scholar of the Leukemia Society of America.

Cr RT and IT MTX have an observed average IQ 13 points lower than expected; (2) the IQ deficit is greatest in those patients who are the youngest when started on leukemia treatment [4, 7, 9].

The primary inciting factor in the pathogenesis of these deficits is probably an adverse interaction between Cr RT and IT MTX [3]. Contributing iatrogenic factors may include intramuscular asparaginase, now known to predispose to cerebral thrombosis and hemorrhage [10], and intravenous vincristine *[Bleyer,* case report of cortical hemorrhage presented at the symposium].

In a study of adolescents with cancer histories, the California Division of The American Cancer Society found that 51% experience cancer-related problems upon their return to school. Nearly half experienced loss of friends, isolation, lack of motor coordination, or speech impairment, and 43% had to eliminate, reduce, or change participation in extra-curricular activities. While some had to withdraw from active sports, others withdrew from activities such as drama, debating and music because of appearance, low energy, or depression.

Heart

Above cumulative doses of 550 mg/m², both daunomycin and adriamycin are more likely to induce congestive heart failure (CHF) in children than in adults <40 years of age [12, 13]. In a study of 5,613 patients administered daunomycin, the CHF dose-response curve was much steeper in 2,861 children (<15 years of age) than in 2,752 adults (>15 years of age) [12].

Liver

Chronic hepatic disease after cancer chemotherapy during childhood is a rare sequelae [6, 8, 11]. Of 369 5-year survivors of childhood cancer, only 2 were found by the LESG to have evidence for chronic liver disease [8].

Kidney

In 7 children completing 3 or more years of maintenance therapy for ALL, renal biopsies revealed only mild toxic effects, which were not associated with elevated BUN or serum creatinine levels [6]. Our own experience with high-dose MTX and cisplatin suggests that children are more likely than adults to recover from the nephrotoxicity of these drugs.

Gonads

Normal gonadal development was observed in 14 boys with ALL who had been treated for 3 years with average cumulative doses of vincristine, 80 mg/m², prednisone, 40,000 mg/m², MTX, 2000 mg/m², and 6MP, 60,000 mg/m² [2]. All patients demonstrated normal Tanner staging, LH, FSH and testosterone levels throughout the course of follow-up (0.2–8.5 years after discontinuation of chemotherapy) [2]. On the other hand, both germ-cell and Leydig-cell dysfunction can occur in adolescents *during* chemotherapy [11]. *Pre*pubertal boys and girls seem relatively resistant to these effects of combination chemotherapy [2, 11].

To date, the most comprehensive study of fetal effects is the National Cancer Institute's experience reported by *Blatt* et al. [1]. 28 children were born to 28 (21 females and 7 males) of 418 patients previously administered intensive chemotherapy at childbearing age. Spontaneous abortions occurred in only two pregnancies. Prenatal exposures included vincristine in 24, prednisone in 16, MTX in 12, cyclophosphamide in 11, 6MP in 7, nitrogen mustard in 7, adriamycin in 7, procarbazine in 6, ara-C in 5, daunomycin in 4, BCNU in 3 and 6TG in 2. Of the 23 females, 19 conceived 1 month to 9 years (median 4 years) after all chemotherapy was stopped, and 4 became pregnant while on chemotherapy (2 during the first 2 months of gestation, 1 during the second trimester, 1 during the third trimester). All 28 live births were normal term infants who have had normal growth and development during a median follow-up of 2.5 years. 1 child has had uncomplicated febrile seizures. No major abnormalities have been observed. Minor anomalies were detected in 3 infants: capillary nevus, pilonidal dimples without spina bifida, and congenital hip dysplasia [1].

Lymphatic Tissue

Children who were <5 years of age at the time of diagnosis have shown a lesser degree of immunosuppression after long-term chemotherapy compared with those who were >5 years of age [5].

Oncogenic Late Effects

The LESG has now registered 200 childhood cancer victims who later developed a second malignant neoplasm. Only 11 (5.5%) had no known genetic predisposition to cancer and had received only chemotherapy such that radiation could not be invoked as an etiologic agent

[8]. Hence, *chemotherapy*-induced neoplasms do not appear to be a major late effect of cancer chemotherapy during childhood, the vast majority being attributable to radiation and/or genetic factors.

Conclusion

On balance, children generally tolerate both the adverse and late effects of cancer chemotherapy better than adults. Exceptions are the neurotoxic sequelae of MTX and CNS irradiation [3], and anthracycline-induced cardiomyopathy [12, 13]. Safer chemotherapeutic regimens are indicated provided that the excellent results currently being achieved with the curative therapies of childhood cancer are maintained. Whether future drugs, drug combination and multimodal therapies will increase the risk of late effects remains to be ascertained. While continuing surveillance is paramount, delayed tragedies have detracted minimally from the current triumphs of cancer therapy in children.

References

1 Blatt, J.; Mulvihill, J.J.; Ziegler, J.L.; Young, R.C.; Poplack, D.G.: Teratogenicity of cancer chemotherapy. Am. J. Med. *69:*828–832 (1980)

2 Blatt, J.; Poplack, D.G.; Sherins, R.J.: Testicular function in boys after chemotherapy for acute lymphoblastic leukemia. New Engl. J. Med. *304:*1121–1124 (1981)

3 Bleyer, W.A.; Griffin, T.W.: White matter necrosis, mineralizing microangiopathy, and intellectual abilities in survivors of childhood leukemia; associations with central nervous system irradiation and methotrexate therapy; in Gilbert, Kagan, Radiation damage to the nervous system, pp. 115–174 (Raven Press, New York 1980)

4 Eiser, C.: Intellectual abilities among survivors of childhood leukaemia as a function of CNS irradiation. Archs Dis. Childh. *53:*391–395 (1978)

5 Haghbin, M.; Cunningham-Rundles, S.; Thaler, H.T.; Gupta, S.; Hecht, S.; Murphy, M.L.; Oettgen, H.F.: Immunotherapy with oral BCG and serial immune evaluation in childhood lymphoblastic leukemia following three years of chemotherapy. Cancer *46:*2577–2586 (1980)

6 Mahoney, D.H.; Gonzales, E.T.; Ferry, G.D.; Sanjad, S.A.; Noorden, G.K. van; Fernbach, D.J.: Systemic side effects of chemotherapy in children with acute leukemia in long term remissions. Blood *54:*suppl. 1, pp. 196 (1979)

7 Meadows, A.T.; Gordon, J.; Littman, P.; Glaser, K.M.; Fergusson, J.: Patterns in children with ALL treated with cranial radiation. Proc. Am. Ass. Cancer Res. Am. Soc. clin. Oncol. *21:*386 (1980)

8 Meadows, A.T.; Krejmas, N.L.; Belasco, J.B.: The medical cost of cure. Sequelae in survivors of childhood cancer; in Eys van, Sullivan, Status of the curability of childhood cancers, pp. 263–272 (Raven Press, New York 1980)

9   Moss, H.A.; Nannis, E.D.; Poplack, D.G.: The effects of prophylactic treatment of
     the central nervous system on the intellectual functioning of children with acute
     lymphocytic leukemia. Am. J. Med. *71*:47–52 (1981).
10   Priest, J.R.; Ramsay, N.K.C.; Latchaw, R.R.; Lockman, L.A.; Hasegawa, D.K.;
     Coates, T.D.; Coccia, P.F.; Edson, J.R.; Nesbit, M.E.; Krivit, W.: Thrombotic and
     hemorrhagic strokes complicating early therapy for childhood acute lymphoblastic
     leukemia. Cancer *46*:1548–1554 (1980)
11   Sherins, R.J.; Olweny, C.L.M.; Ziegler, J.L.: Gynecomastia and gonadal dysfunc-
     tion in adolescent boys treated with combination chemotherapy for Hodgkin's dis-
     ease. New Engl. J. Med. *299*:12–16 (1978)
12   Hoff, D.D. von; Rozencweig, M.; Layard, M.; Slavik, M.; Muggio, F.M.: Dauno-
     mycin-induced cardiotoxicity in children and adults. Am. J. Med. *62:* 200–208
     (1977)
13   Hoff, D.D. von; Layard, M.W.; Basa, P.; Davis, H.L.; Hoff, A.L. von; Rozencweig,
     M.; Muggio, F.M.: Risk factors for adriamycin-induced congestive heart failure.
     Ann. intern. Med. *91*:710–717 (1979).

W.A. Bleyer, MD, Children's Orthopedic Hospital and Medical Center,
University of Washington, Fred Hutchinson Cancer Research Center,
Seattle, WA 98105 (USA)

Front. Radiat. Ther. Onc., vol. 16, pp. 55–61 (Karger, Basel 1982)

Individualized Patient Chemotherapy: Use of a Human Tumor Colony Formation Technique[1]

Frank L. Meyskens, Jr.[2]

Department of Internal Medicine and Cancer Center Division, University of Arizona, Tucson, Ariz., USA

Introduction

Rationale

De novo and acquired resistance of human cancer cells to chemotherapy is a common problem in oncology. Various in vitro and in vivo methods have been used to identify useful drugs against human tumors [2]. Most of these assays depend on the general antiproliferative effect of chemotherapeutic agents in tissue culture lines or transplantable tumors which have become clonally selected over time and do not consider the clonal heterogeneity that is present in most naturally occurring tumors. This concept is diagrammatically represented in figure 1.

Development of Tumor Clonogenic Assay

Studies of normal murine and human hematopoietic cells have shown that a small subpopulation of primitive cells give rise to all subsequent precursors [7]. A similar group of cells has been identified in human myeloid leukemia [1]. These cells are called stemcells, and the early progeny is designated progenitor or clonogenic cells (fig. 1). Recently a technique was developed by *Hamburger and Salmon* [3] to grow clonogenic cells from human tumors. In this system only malignant colony-forming cells proliferate. After 7- to 14-day colonies arising from a single cell can be enumerated. A photomicrograph of a melanoma colony is shown in figure 2.

[1] The author thanks *M. Henley, B. Soehnlen,* and *L. Young* for technical assistance and *S. Salmon* for his continued assistance in this work.

[2] Supported in part by Public Health Service Grants.

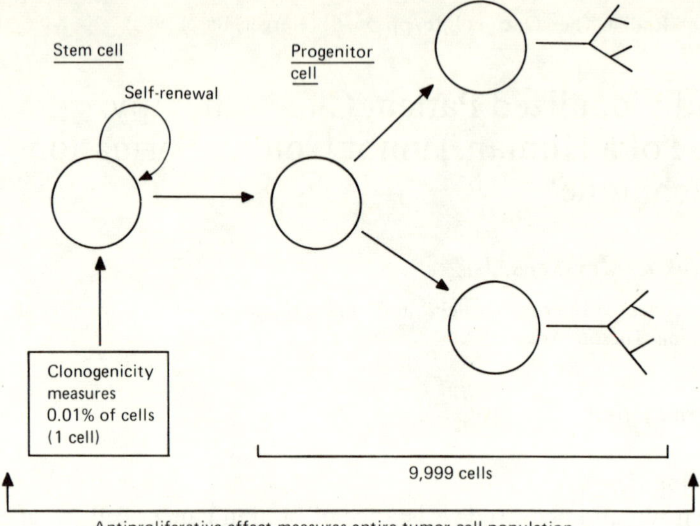

Fig. 1. Measurement of the effect of drugs on clonogenicity versus proliferation.

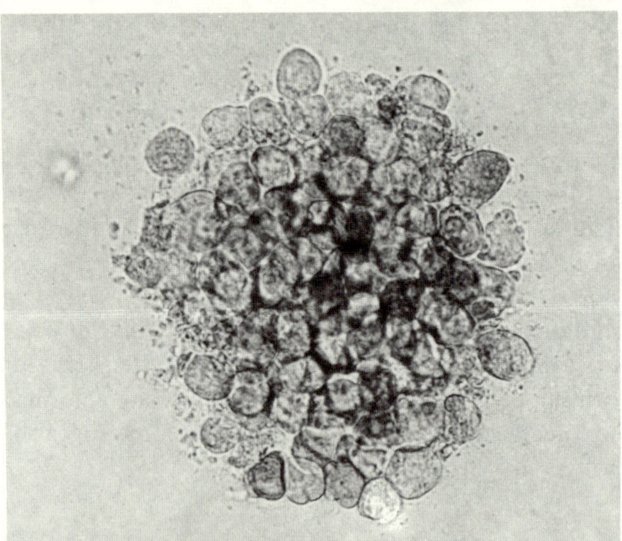

Fig. 2. Melanoma colony 10 days after plating of suspension of single tumor cells. ×200

Table I. Requirements for an in vitro chemotherapy drug testing system

1	Must be technically simple and/or readily automated
2	Should be adaptable to a wide variety of tumors
3	A substantial (one log or greater) kill should be readily detectable
4	A wide variety of different chemotherapeutic agents should be testable in the system
5	The concentration of drug used in vitro should be pharmacologically achievable in vivo
6	In vitro drug effect should be reflected in in vivo clinical response

Clonogenic assays for several human tumors [8] including ovarian carcinoma [5], multiple myeloma [4], and malignant melanoma [6] have been reported.

Requirements for an in vitro Predictive Assay

If an assay is to be useful in a predictive screening mode, it should fulfill the criteria outlined in table I.

Many systems have fulfilled the first five requirements, but the sine qua non for a predictive assay that will influence individual patient chemotherapy is that in vitro sensitivity and resistance must accurately correlate with clinical response.

In vitro/in vivo Correlations

In vitro/in vivo correlations using the tumor clonogenic assay have been reported for ovarian cancer, multiple myeloma, and melanoma [9, 10]. Clinical resistance was predicted with 95% accuracy overall and clinical response with over 65% precision. The approach used to define in vitro response involves measurement of the area under the curve at one-tenth the pharmacologically achievable concentration and is detailed elsewhere [10]. As a modus operandi we use a 70% decrease in colony survival at pharmacologically achievable concentrations as indicating considerable sensitivity to the drug. In our experience less than a 70% reduction has infrequently resulted in a clinical response. The major patterns of response are shown in figure 3.

Using a 70% reduction in colony survival as an indication of sensitivity we have correlated in vitro effect to clinical response in malig-

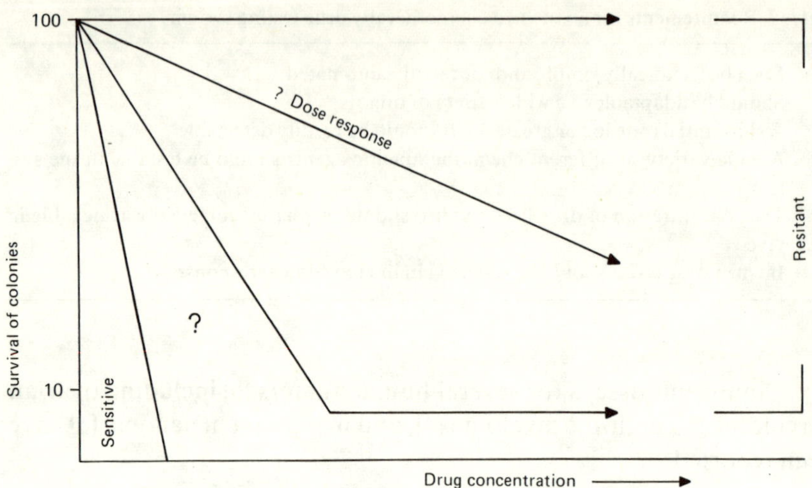

Fig. 3. Patterns of response of tumor clonogenic cells to chemotherapy.

Table II. Correlation of in vitro effect in the clonogenic assay and clinical response (first 24 patients)

	In vivo	
	R	S
In vitro		
R	88%	12%
S	52%	48%

R = Resistance; S = sensitivity.

nant melanoma. These results are summarized in table II. Resistance was predicted with high frequency (88%), comparable to that seen in multiple myeloma and ovarian cancer [10]. Sensitivity was predicted with 48% accuracy. This precision is somewhat less than that seen for ovarian cancer and myeloma, but still at least three times better than if agents were used blindly. The lower precision in predicting sensitivity with melanoma than in ovarian cancer or multiple myeloma may be related to either extensive clonal heterogeneity in melanoma and/or that melanoma clonogenic cells must be exquisitely sensitive to drugs in vitro for a clinical response to be detected. The presence of a high

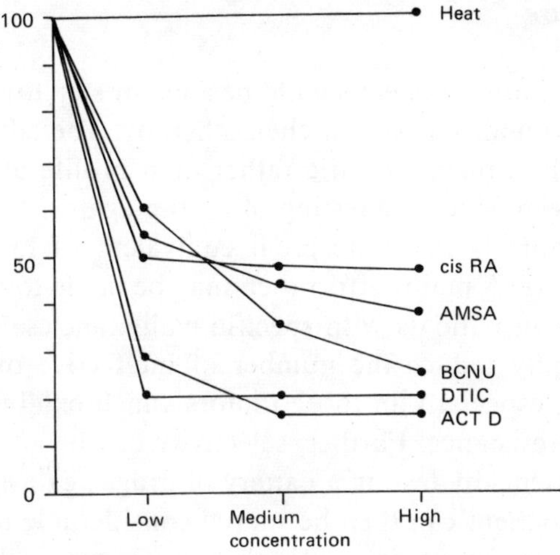

Fig. 4. Multiple drug testing in an individual patient.

incidence of both false positive and false negative correlation in melanoma argue for tumor heterogeneity as playing an important role. This can be tested by examining for drug sensitivity in several nodules in the same patient at the same time. Our preliminary studies suggest that extensive biological and chemotherapeutic heterogeneity do exist. The alternative possibility of the necessity of exquisite sensitivity in vitro will be examined by testing the effect of lower concentrations of drugs in future patients.

Individualized Patient Chemotherapy

An example of the potential usefulness in this system is demonstrated in figure 4. This particular patient had been previously treated with BCG, melphalan,. and hydroxyurea. Six modalities were tested. In vitro, four agents exhibited little activity at pharmacologically achievable (low) doses, and thusly the patient would not receive these ineffective drugs. DTIC and actinomycin D appeared to reduce colony survival at low concentrations. The patient received this drug and experienced a complete response of multiple subcutaneous nodules and a partial response of lung nodules within 1 month which has been sustained for 4 months.

Thoughts for the Future

The tumor clonogenic assay system should be a major step toward tumor-specific and individualized patient chemotherapy. The advantages of any assay which is *tumor*-specific rather than proliferation-specific can be readily seen, since the testing of a drug against 5 random transplantable tumors is the conceptual equivalent of testing tumor cells from 5 patients. A major effort then may be made toward using only certain drugs in patients with specific malignancies. This stratagem should markedly reduce the number of ineffective drugs used in specific cancers, especially in those tumors which exhibit de novo chemotherapeutic resistance. Further, selectivity can be accomplished in individual patients by testing a battery of drugs against the own tumor (fig. 4). The patient can then be spared considerable morbidity by not receiving ineffective drugs. Further, drugs with a high probability of success can be selected and used.

Other expectations and possibilities of the clonogenic assay as a tool to understanding human tumor biology are detailed elsewhere [9], but the technique has already generated sufficient interest that large scale testing of the validity of this approach have begun and appear promising.

References

1   Buick, R.N.; Till, J.E.; McCulloch, E.A.: Colony assay for proliferative blast cells circulating in myeloblastic leukemia. Lancet *1*:862 (1977)
2   Dendy, P.P.: Human tumors in short term culture: techniques and clinical applications (Academic Press, New York, 1976)
3   Hamburger, A.W.; Salmon, S.E.: Primary bioassay of human tumor stem cells. Science *197*:461 (1977)
4   Hamburger, A.W.; Salmon, S.E.: Primary biossay of human tumor stem cells. J. clin. Invest. *60*:846 (1977)
5   Hamburger, A.W.; Salmon, S.E.; Kim, M.B.: Direct cloning of human ovarian carcinoma cells in agar. Cancer Res. *38*:3438 (1978)
6   Meyskens, F.L.; Salmon, S.E.: Inhibition of human melanoma colony formation by retinoids. Cancer Res. *39*:4055 (1979)
7   McCulloch, E.A.; Buick, R.N.; Till, J.E.: Cellular differentiation in the myeloblastic leukemias of man; in Saunders, Cell differentiation and neoplasia (Raven Press, New York 1978)
8   Salmon, S.E.: Human tumor cloning in vitro (Liess, New York in press 1980)

9   Salmon, S.E.; Alberts, D.S.; Durie, B.G.M.; Meyskens, F.L.; Jones, S.E.; Soehnlen, B.; Chen, H.S.G.; Moon, T.E.: Clinical correlations of drug sensitivity in the human tumor stem cell assay; in Recent results in cancer research (Springer, New York 1979)

10   Salmon, S.E.; Hamburger, A.W.; Soehnlen, B.J.; Meyskens, F.L.; Jones, S.E.; Soehnlen, B.; Chen. H.S.G.; Moon, T.E.: Quantitation of differential sensitivity of human tumor stem cells to anticancer drugs. New Engl. J. med. *298*: 1321 (1978).

F.L. Meyskens, Jr., MD, Department of Internal Medicine, and
Cancer Center Division, University of Arizona, Tucson, AZ 85724 (USA)

Front. Radiat. Ther. Onc., vol. 16, pp. 62–82 (Karger, Basel 1982)

Radiation Sensitivity and Organ Tolerances in Pediatric Oncology: A New Hypothesis

Philip Rubin, Paul Van Houtte, Louis Constine

Division of Radiation Oncology, University of Rochester, Cancer Center, Rochester, N.Y., USA

The child, like the embryo, is a mosaic of numerous tissues and organs which are undergoing continual growth and maturation. These tissues and organs have cells that are in various stages of development: totipotential, multipotential, and eventually unipotential which are either resting or in active proliferation without or with differentiation into specialized tissues or organs. Just as the fetus in its development is continually changing in its tissue and cellular kinetics, so in turn is its radiosensitivity with critical points in time of exquisite vulnerability to irradiation for specific organs. Similarly, the infant and child consist of an array of tissues and organs that vary in radiosensitivity at different times according to their developmental stage.

The hypothesis advanced for understanding the changing radiosensitivity and radioresistance of pediatric tissues is in comprehending their periods of active proliferation and differentiation and eventual maturation. Growth of an organ varies from infancy, childhood and puberty and is not constant. Correction factors applied for radiation dose are modified by age but do not recognize that various organs indeed develop and mature at different rates (table I). No one formula can be applied universally to all tissues.

Adjusted doses for age assumes that growth occurs at a constant rate. The growth rate and maturation of each tissue or organ is the major determinant of its radiosensitivity. A model for pediatric radiosensitivity of normal tissues and organs is developed in an analogous fashion to fetal organ radiosensitivity.

Table I. Dose corrections by age for infradiaphragmatic sides

0–12 months	1,200–1,800 rad
13–18 months	1,801–2,400 rad
19–30 months	2,401–3,000 rad
31–40 months	3,001–3,500 rad
>41 months	3,501–4,000 rad

National Wilms' tumor study for unfavorable histology.

The Fetal Model of Radiosensitivity: Prenatal Organogenesis

The susceptibility of the fetus to radiation and the resultant dramatic occurrence of congenital abnormalities has been the subject of intense study. Analogies have been drawn between experimental studies in mammalian fetal radiobiology and abnormalities observed in human circumstances. It is possible to extrapolate from these laboratory studies to man.

The principle events in the development of an embryo include implantation, placentation, organogenesis, and differentiation of the various organs. The sequence of events tends to be the same in different mammalian species with only the time scale differing [11, 16, 36]. Both in the experimental model and in clinical experience, moderate doses of ionizing radiation have been shown to produce catastrophic effects in the fetus which include growth retardation, fetal death, or gross congenital malformation [36]. In the mouse, a dose of 200 rad will lead to prenatal deaths in the preimplantation phases, abnormalities or neonatal deaths during the organogenesis (fig. 1) [38]. Neural tissues are interestingly the most exquisitely sensitive and most rapidly dividing in early fetal development. An exposure of 100–500 rad during the course of embryogenesis suffices to produce neural malformations, mainly an overall reduction of brain size as micro-opthalmy or micro–cephaly [16]. In comparison, 2 weeks after birth, doses greater than 1,000 rad are necessary to produce neurologic abnormalities in rats [9, 52]. Information available from Japanese survivors of the A bomb attacks show an increase in fetal deaths, infant deaths, and neurologic abnormalities [24]. Doses lower than 250 rad delivered between the 4th and 20th weeks of gestation may lead to severe abnormalities.

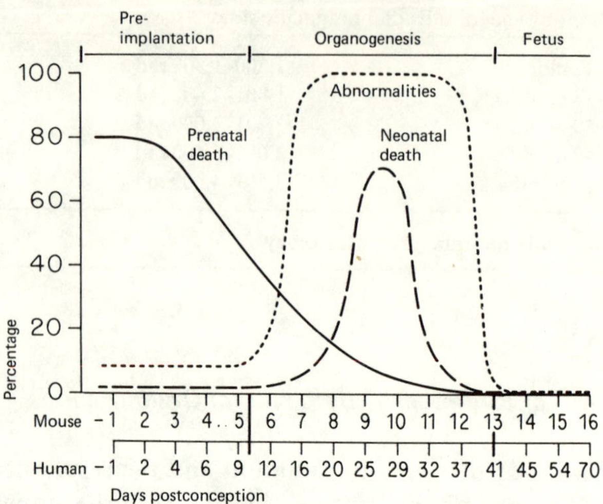

Fig. 1. Incidence of abnormalities and of prenatal and neonatal deaths in mice given a dose of 200 rad at various times after fertilization. The lower scale consists of *Rugh's* estimates of the equivalent stages for the human embryo [from ref. 16].

The Pediatric Model of Radiosensitivity: Postnatal Growth Spurts

Instead of the critical moments, days or weeks for fetal organ induction and rapid development, in the child there are longer periods of months for rapid proliferation when the entire parenchyma of an organ is in a phase of active mitosis. At some point the collective of tissues or cells becomes mature and differentiates into a specialized system. Some systems have rapid proliferation or cell cycle kinetic characteristics whereas others behave as slow renewal systems and only become active again if challenged or stimulated. 'When does a pediatric tissue or organ become similar to an adult tissue or organ?' is a question that needs to be answered. Postnatal development has been studied much less than prenatal development and information on variation in growth characteristics are less well known.

In the child, there are two major periods of rapid rate of growth development: the postnatal period and puberty. The growth of the different organs follows four general patterns (fig. 2) [14, 42–44]. The first is a general skeletal pattern which has the two peak periods aforementioned. The organs of circulation and digestion follow the pattern of the body as a whole (postnatal and pubertal activity). The neural type

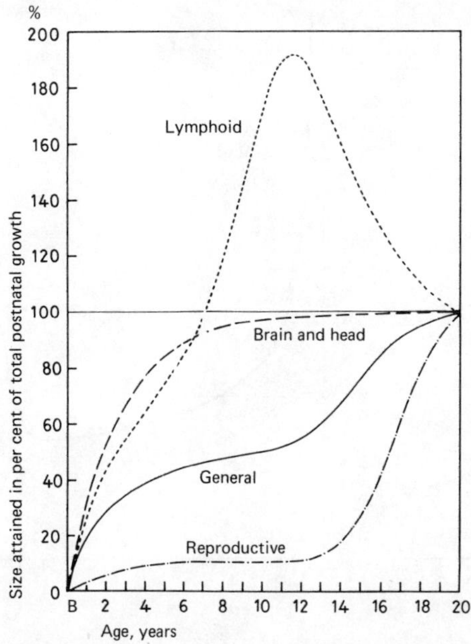

Fig. 2. Growth curves of different parts and tissues of the body, showing the four chief types. All the curves are of size attained, and plotted as percent of total gain from birth to 20 years, so that size at age 20 is 100 on the vertical scale [from ref. 42].

is characterized by a rapid postnatal growth which slows in late infancy and ceases in adolescence. The respiratory and renal organs tend to follow this pattern according to their maturation. The genital type shows little change during early life but rapid development just before and coincident with puberty. This is particularly true of breast tissue and applies to testis and ovarian tissue. The lymphoid type is characterized by a gradual evolution and involution to the time of puberty.

A number of different organs will be reviewed regarding their growth maturation and radiosensitivity for the different stages of proliferation and differentation. Organ weight and size may be helpful guides, but it is essential to determine when an organ is through or is entering its phase of rapid proliferation. It is important to distinguish hyperplasia from hypertrophy as to the mechanism of organ growth. To fully understand an organ's radiosensitivity it is necessary first to comprehend its biology.

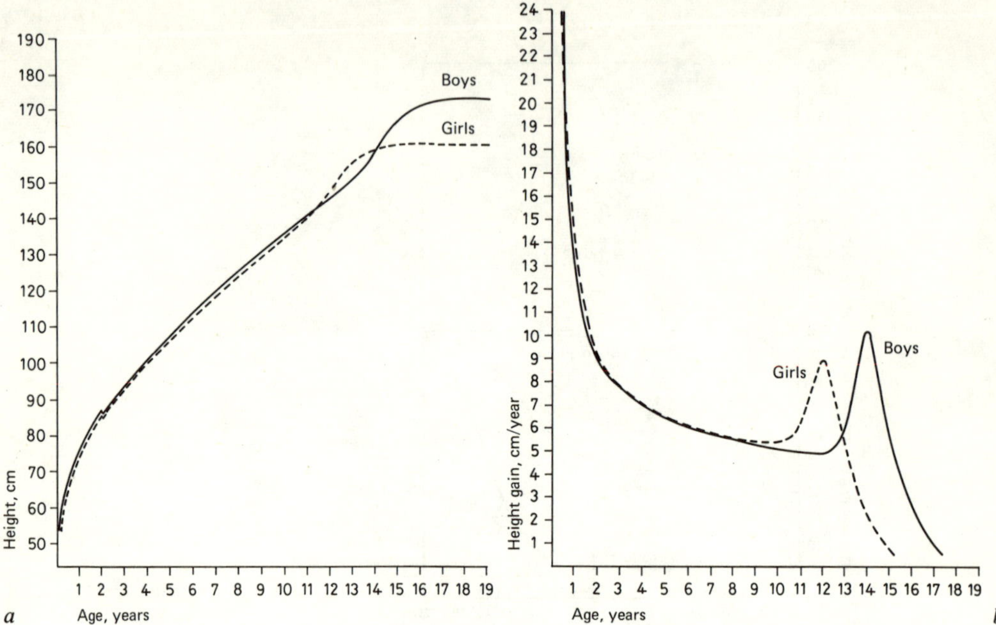

Fig. 3. a Typical-individual height-attained curves for boys and girls (supine length to the age of 2) [from ref. 43]. *b* Typical-individual velocity curves for supine length or height in boys and girls. These curves represent the velocity of the typical boy and girl at any given instant. [from ref. 43].

General Type or Skeletal Growth

Bone growth is not a uniform process in either time or spatially in regard to skeletal development. Rapid growth occurs postnatally and then prior to and during puberty with a period of steady growth from 5 to 10 years of age (fig. 3) [43]. The process of growth in individual bones varies and depends upon whether it is a long bone, a short bone, a cuboid bone or a flat bone. There are two processes that shape each bone: intramembranous and endochondral bone formation. Bone length, which determines body size, is a function of cartilage growth or endochondral bone. Longitudinal growth is due to rapid proliferation of chondroblasts that in turn are replaced by invading vessels. The mucopolysaccharide/chondrotin ground substance is remodeled into osteoid and bone by osteoblasts and osteoclasts. Bone width is a function of intramembranous bone growth and is also a life-long remodeling process which is determined by muscle pull and weight bearing [21,

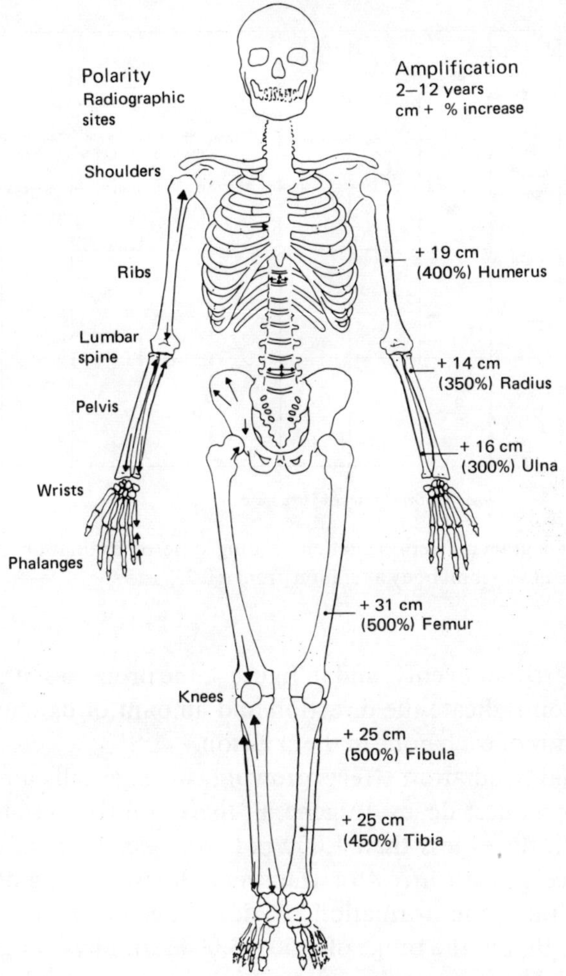

Fig. 4. The rate and direction of growth at specific skeletal sites are indicated by the length and thickness of the arrows. *Amplification* is the concept that the bone showing the greatest growth potential will show the greatest change, since it will magnify the same defect to a greater degree. *Polarity* is the concept that tubular bones grow in a differential pattern, with one end predominating over the other. The maximal direction of longitudinal growth is its polarity. *Time* is the scale against which the severity of the defect in modeling is measured [from ref. 35].

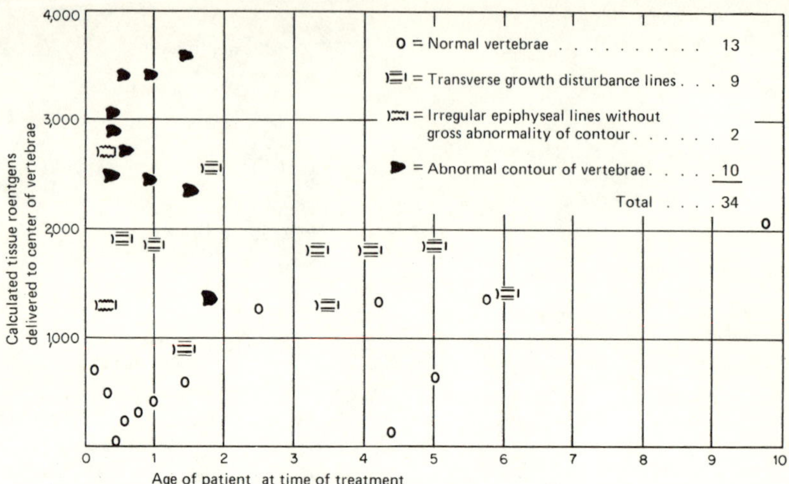

Fig. 5. Diagramatic representation relating dose of irradiation and age of the patient to type of vertebral body alteration [from ref. 25].

35]. Bones grow unevenly, and in figure 4, the processes of polarity and amplification indicate the direction and amount of osseous growth at different ends of each bone in the skeleton.

External irradiation effects growing cartilage cells and bone cells with rather modest doses. In general, there is little alteration in bone growth with doses less than 1,000 rad, whereas doses of 1,000–2,000 rad produce growth arrest or transverse lines. To completely arrest endochondral bone formation, a dose greater than 2,000 rad is required so that in the range of 2,500–3,000 rad, physical growth stops completely. Location of the most rapidly growing epiphyseal plate is important to determine if the placement of the field will produce severe stunting, e.g., proximal versus distal epiphysis in the humerus and femurs, respectively. This seems to be modified by age but can be illusory in that the early arrest of bone growth produces a greater stunting effect than a later arrest. The radiosensitivity of cells is the same but the greater reduction in growth is inherent in the biologic age of the event rather than reflecting an altered radiosensitivity of chondroblasts with age [12, 45].

In the 'classic' study of *Neuhauser* et al. [25], 45 patients treated for intra-abdominal tumors at ages between 4 months to 9 years developed

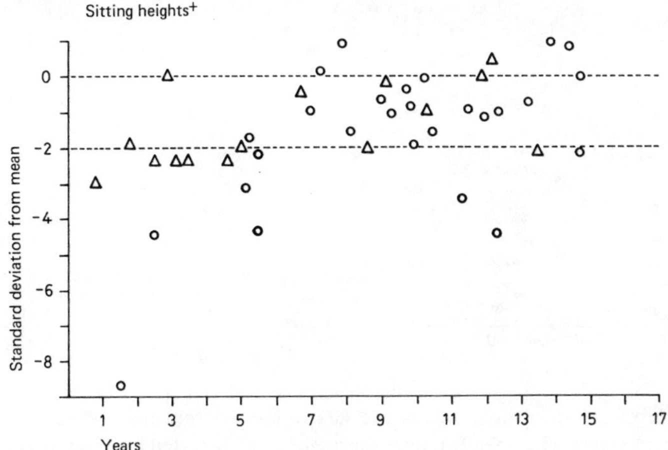

Fig. 6. Variation from normal sitting height of children irradiated to the spinal axis for medulloblastoma, Hodgkin's disease or ALL related to the dose delivered; △<2,500 rads; ○>3,500 rads [from ref. 32].

severe changes. These occurred as a function of age and dose so that patients less than 2 years old and doses greater than 2,000 rad produced the most pronounced deformities (fig. 5). *Probert and Parker* [32] measured the standing and sitting height of children irradiated for Hodgkin's disease, medulloblastoma, and acute lymphoblastic leukemia (ALL). The reduction in sitting height reflected the amount of vertebral irradiation these children received and proved to be both dose- and age-dependent. The retardation of spinal growth was seen in children irradiated during the periods of most active growth, i.e., under 6 years of age and during puberty (fig. 6). *Tefft* [45] similarly concluded that children under 1 year of age at the time of irradiation had roentgenographic changes with 300 ret while more than 1,000 ret were necessary to induce significant effects in children beyond 2 years of age. The decrease in sitting height, as noted by *Probert and Parker* [32], was with doses beyond 3,500 rad and was less visible with doses less than 2,500 rad.

A recent survey and analysis of postirradiation slipped epiphysis indicates again a clear relationship to dose and age. A specific threshold dose is required, i.e., >2,500 rad to produce this phenomenon and it occurs (table II, fig. 7) in 50% of children less than 4 years (7/15) as

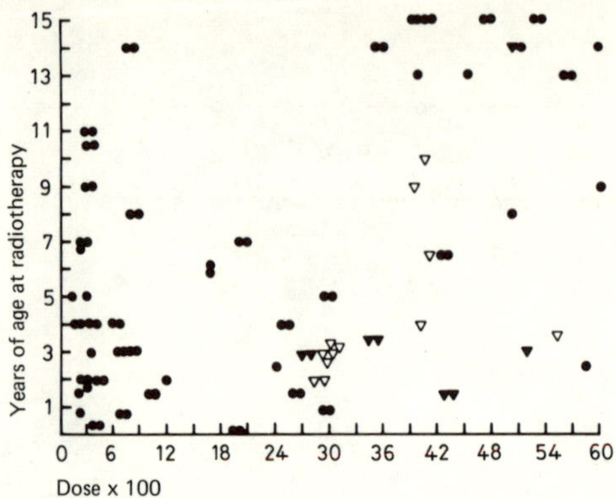

Fig. 7. Relationship of dose versus age at irradiation from the normal and the affected physical plates. The open triangles represent cases reported by *Wolf, Ryan and Chapman;* ▽ = Cases, ▼ = slipped epiphysis or severe abnormalities; ● = normal epiphysis [from ref. 40].

Table II. Incidence of slipped epiphysis by age and dose; from *Silverman* et al. [40]

	0–2 years	2–4 years	4–10 years	10–15 years
≤2,500 rad	0/14	0/11	0/16	0/6
>2,500 rad	4/8	3/7	0/6	1/15

compared to only 1/21 with older children ranging from 5 to 15 years. The slippage occurred at around 8–10 years of age independent of time of irradiation and the authors suggest it could be due to the increased tilting of this femoral line. Another time of vulnerability is preceding puberty due to rapid growth expressing the radiation-induced abnormality [40].

In contrast to pediatric bone, in adult bone large doses are required to produce osteonecrosis. Even with doses >5,000 rad, osteonecrosis rarely occurs and is more common with orthovoltage irradiation due to greater energy absorption. Rarely does the circumstance exist in adults for bone growth to be effected except as a remodeling process. When fractures occur, endochondral bone process is a vital part of callous formation, but this event is blocked with rather modest radiation doses, recapitulating the pediatric sensitivity of growing bone and cartilage to irradiation [27].

The Neural Type of Growth: Brain

The brain is most exquisitely sensitive from its prenatal organogenesis in the first trimester of gestation and throughout the remaining early postnatal period when it increases in size [11, 16]. In the first year of life, there is rapid increase in the cranial vault compared to the facial bones since the skull dimensions are related to the rapid increase in size of the brain [5, 18]. By the 6 year, the growth has slowed and the brain in children is similar in size to adults. The period of organogenesis is the period of exquisite radiosensitivity with doses of >15 rad producing nervous system abnormalities in rodents as microcephaly and enencephaly [36]. Once the central nervous system is developed in utero, the number of neurons are fixed and overall brain size is mainly due to an increase in size, not numbers of cells. This system is a fixed renewal system in which neurons are long lived and have lost their ability to replicate.

In brief, the development of the brain comprizes the following phases: neural plate development, neuroblast proliferation, glial cell proliferation, axon migration, synapse formation with myelinization. The neuronal cell division occurs prenatally and the glial cell proliferation is largely a postnatal event with a peak of replication at 3 months of age; the growth in DNA contents continues into the second year (time of plateau is approximately 18 months) [4, 13]. If the full maturation is judged by the degree of myelinization, this is not reached until puberty or later. However, this process is at least well advanced in most regions by the end of the second year [51].

Studies on rats show a direct relation between doses of irradiation, age and toxicity for the first 2 weeks of life. During this period DNA content is still increasing and reaches a plateau after 2 weeks. After the 5th day there is marked decrease in the incidence and the severity of the neurologic signs even for doses of 1,000 rad. Radiation after the 15th day resulted in no visible neurologic findings even for a single dose of 1,000 rad (fig. 8) [9, 52]. Irradiation damage to brain in children is difficult to evaluate precisely as neurologic deficiencies may be the result of the space-occupying lesion, surgery or combined treatments. Radiation doses have been usually reduced in children younger than 3 years. This limit has been chosen as the size of the brain is then 75% of the adult. Nevertheless, the exact tolerance of a child's brain has not been precisely defined and this limit is quite arbitrary [3, 19].

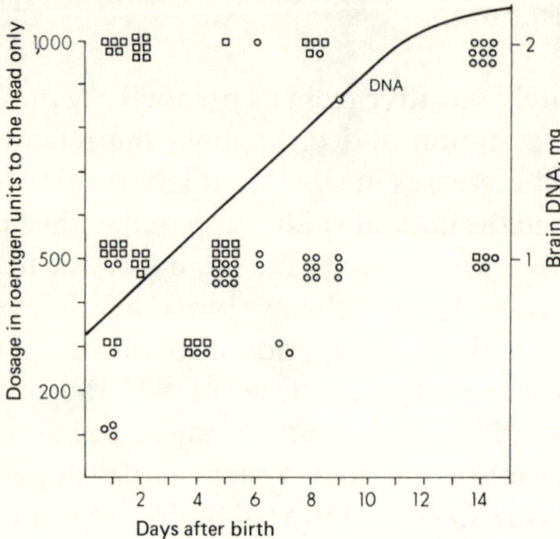

Fig. 8. Graphs showing the production of neurologic signs by head irradiation (one single fraction) in the neonatal rat related to age and to DNA growth curve; □ = pathologic CNS signs; O = no pathologic CNS signs [from ref. 52].

The Genital Type of Growth: Breast

Some tissues or organs are quiescent during infancy and childhood until puberty. Rapid stimulus to general skeletal growth occurs at this time and then ceases. The breast is an excellent example of genital growth with no growth during infancy and childhood and then a rapid increase in size only at puberty. Irradiation of the infantile breast inhibits development of the mammary gland and doses of 500–1,000 rad induce later hypoplasia and aplasia. By contrast, the adult breast tolerates high doses with minimal change up to 5,000–6,000 rad, doses used in treating early breast cancer with excellent cosmesis. Gynecomastia can be prevented in male adults receiving estrogen therapy for prostate cancer by prior irradiation to a modest dose of 1,000–2,000 rad whereas similar doses are ineffective if given after the induction of breast tissue proliferation.

Unclassified: Lung

Many organs have not been fully classified as to their growth kinetics which include periods of proliferation, periods of hypertrophy, and a period of maturation. Alveolar formation begins during the end

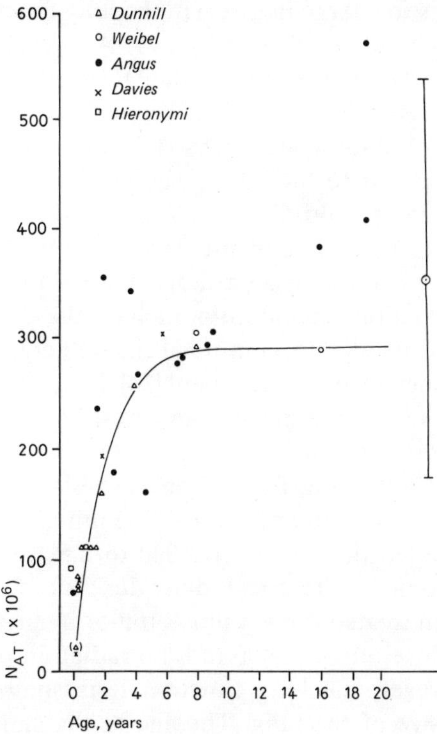

Fig. 9. The total number of alveoli (N_{AT}) found in the lung as reported by several observers is plotted against age. The adult range found by *Angus* and *Thurlbeck* is shown at the right. The solid line is the regression line calculated by *Dunnill* from his data [ref. 46].

of the fetal life and continues postnatally. While most investigators agree that the majority of alveoli appear in the postnatal period, the time at which alveolar multiplication ceases is much disputed from 1 year to the end of the growth spurt. However, most authors believe that the most rapid phase of pulmonary growth or alveolar multiplication and cellular proliferation occur in the first months of life, certainly within the first year, and then are followed by a period of slow growth of alveolarization of bronchioles within 4–6 years postnatally (fig. 9). Later, alveolar surface increases mainly by an increase in volume or size, not number [17, 46]. Radiographic measurements of the lung diameters shows a linear growth during childhood with a spurt at puberty [41]. This corresponds to a large increase in the lung functions except for the resistance which falls as the child grows. As it is always hazardous to translate animal data to the human, the DNA increase of the lung in the rat follows closely the curves of the brain and reaches a plateau after 2 weeks of life [46]. Within a few days after birth the structure of the alveoli appears similar to the adult. The vascular system grows in parallel with the alveolar multiplication. Therapeutic irradiation to the lung in children can either limit the development of new alveoli or produce radiation pneumonitis. Variables known to influence the development of radiation pneumonitis include the dose of irradiation, the volume of lung irradiated, combined chemotherapeutic agents and the presence of a metastatic involvement [34]. Irradiation of the growing cartilage and bones of the thorax can arrest its development and in turn limit the size of the lung.

The data available for whole lung irradiation suggests that the level of tolerance is similar for children and adults. The initial reports of *Newton and Spittle* [26] noted that doses of 2,000 to 2,500 rad in adults produces fatal pneumonitis at fractional daily doses of 150 rad. In two small series of children treated for a Wilms's tumor by prophylactic lung irradiation with doses under 1,400 rad, no radiation pneumonitis was observed. However, the lung function tests showed a decrease in the subsequent size of the lung. The age of the children ranged from 1½ to 10 years with an average age of 4 years [20, 50].

From recent analysis of single exposure, there is a slight difference between adult and childhood experiences. Precise dose-response data for adults is reported by *Fryer* et al. [15] with a threshold for pneumonitis starting at 750 rad reaching a 100% incidence at 950–1,000 rad. In leukemia children, the curve is shifted slightly to the right starting at 850 rad, plateauing at 1,200 rad and probably reflects a lower dose rate of delivery. It clearly is not less than the adult level.

Occasional case reports of radiation pneumonitis at levels below 2,000 rad and the recommendation to use lower fractional daily doses than 200 rad indicate that the child lung may be more radiosensitive. However, the evidence is unclear as to whether a real difference in radiation sensitivity exists. This may be compatible with the central role alveolar type II cells play in acute radiation pneumonitis [28, 29, 34]. Since the alveolar type II cell is present in adequate numers at birth and is essential for survival, it may support the similarity in radiosensitivity of the infant, child and adult lung.

Discussion: Combined Effects of Chemotherapy-Radiotherapy on Normal Tissue

In children as in adults, the entire concept of radioresistance of normal tissues has been completely modified by the introduction of the multimodal approach. Treatment optimization by adding several modes (chemotherapy, surgery, etc.) has led to increasing cure rates. However, late effects in patients are occurring after the delivery of 'safe' doses below threshold levels [47]. The additive effects of chemotherapy prior, during or after a course of radiation has modified the patterns of radiation response and side or late effects occur in an unpredictable fashion. This changing of concepts in normal tissue and organ radioresistance will be illustrated by two examples.

Lung

A large numer of drugs have been identified which produce pulmonary complications and include bleomycin, busulfan, chlorambucil, cyclophosphamide, melphalan and BCNU [49]. One of the most intensively studied agents is BCNU which has resulted in severe late pulmonary toxicity and lethality and was discovered unfortunately in surviving brain tumor patients kept on prolonged maintenance drug schedules for months to years [1]. An increase in late pulmonary reactions has been identified when bleomycin, actinomycin D and adriamycin have been added to radiation schedules [8]. The modification in dose has been plotted by *Wara and Phillips* [48] (fig. 10) for children receiving radiation and actinomycin D for Wilms's tumor. A further emphasis on the importance of daily fractionation and concurrent chemotherapy is noted by the same authors. Doses less than 2,000 rad in ten fractions were tolerated but fatal pneumonitis occurred above 2,000 rad and reached a 100% level at 3,000 rad. The tolerable ret doses for whole lung irradiation is less than 800 ret (5% incidence) rapidly rising to a 50% incidence at 1,000 ret. With actinomycin D, the tolerable level is reduced to 750 ret for a TD50/5 maximal tissue tolerance dose associated with a 50% complication rate occurring within 5 years. The masking of radiation lesions by prednisone has been recognized when MOPP programs were combined with intensive chest irradiation for Hodgkin's disease patients [7]. Sudden stoppage of prednisone led to fulminating pneumonopathy and careful tapering of steroids is required. When treating the whole of both lungs and the mediastinum, further dose modification is required [6].

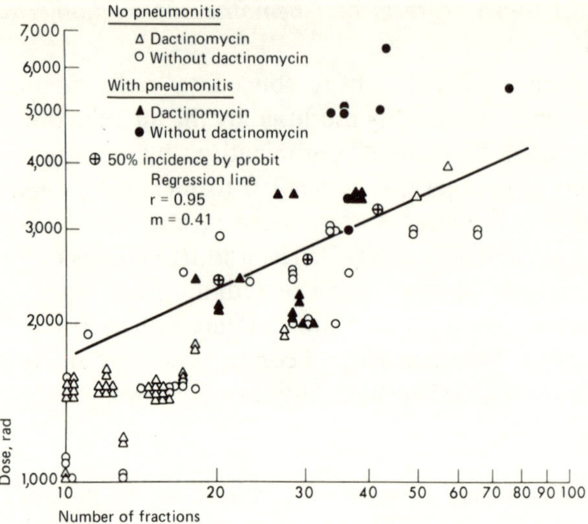

Fig. 10. Radiation combined with dactinomycin produces radiation pneumonitis with much lower doses: there is a 1,000- to 2,000-rad difference between the radiation dose producing pneumonitis with the drug as compared to without it [from ref. 48].

Brain

The treatment for childhood ALL has become very effective in the past decade through the use of multiple-agent chemotherapy and pre-symptomatic central nervous system treatment. Nevertheless, encephalopathies, changes in the intellect and pituitary-hypothalamic dysfunction have been reported with combinations of moderate doses of irradiation, 2,000–2,400 rad, and of methotrexate (MTX) [2, 22, 23, 39].

Studies conducted by the NCI and at Philadelphia among long-term survivors showed a deficit in the intellectual function 3–4 years after treatment; the deficit was greater among children younger than 6 years at diagnosis [23].

In a series of postmortem examinations, the severity of the cerebral atrophy was observed to the intrathecal injection of MTX with or without radiation therapy; the age of the child appears also to influence the results – the younger children presented with the more severe lesion (table III) [10]. Those observations must be related to the cerebral cortex evolution. Between 6 and 8 years, a remodeling of the cortex takes place including decrease in the cortical thickness and in the

Table III. Mean age of onset and duration of illness among children with acute leukemia and cortical atrophy; from *Crosley* et al. [10]

Diagnosis	Degree of cortical atrophy			
	none	mild	moderate	severe
ALL				
Number of patients	22	24	17	5
Age at onset, months	89±52	77±46	68±42	29±24″
Duration, months	20±14	24±16	34±26*	16±8
AML				
Number of patients	10	8	5	0
Age at onset, months	113±48	63±40**	95±46	—
Duration, months	13±11	15±10	17±9	—
Total				
Number of patients	32	32	22	5
Age at onset, months	97±52	74±50*	74±46*	29±24**
Duration, months	17±13	22±16	30±23***	16±8

* p < 0.05; ** p < 0.0025; *** p < 0.01

dendritic pattern and increase in the number of nerve cells in the different layers [33]. The mineralizing microangiopathy with dystrophic calcification was only observed among children younger than 10 years [30], most often in the first 6 years (fig. 11). On the other hand, no precise correlation with age was found for the subacute or the disseminated necrotizing leukoencephalopathy. This complication is fortunately low and its incidence increases when several modalities are combined: intravenous MTX, intrathecal MTX, irradiation. Moreover, increasing doses of MTX or irradiation increases this complication [2, 31].

Conclusions

The following tenets are offered as guidelines to pediatric organ radiosensitivity: (1) The stage of organogenesis, during fetal development when an organ is being formed, is the most highly radiosensitive phase. (2) Specific phases of tissue proliferation during infancy and childhood when rapid growth spurts occur determine the organ's radio-

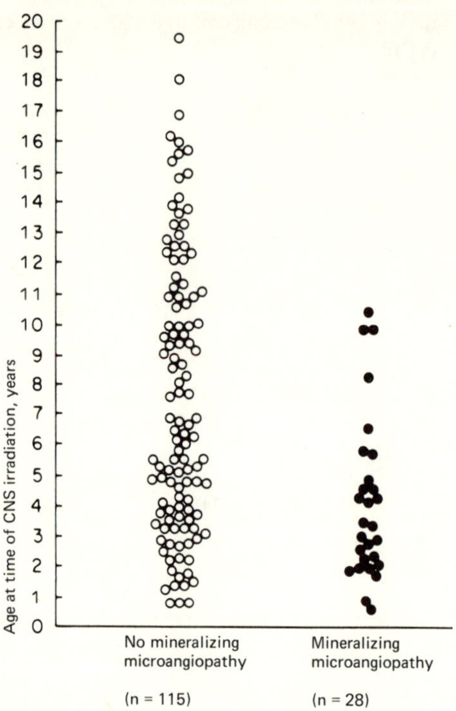

Fig. 11. Association between mineralizing microangiopathy and age at time of cranial irradiation [from ref. 31].

sensitivity. Radiosensitivity of a tissue/organ is highest prior to and at the time of onset of proliferative activity in each organ system. (3) Maturation occurs at different ages for each tissue/organ and its identification allows for recognition when the radiosensitivity in children is similar to adults. (4) Growth of an organ due to increase in cell size is less vulnerable to irradiation than when due to an increase in cell number, i.e., hypertrophy versus proliferation. (5) Radiation therapy and chemotherapy can be additive even when safe schedules are given and can lead to late effects despite intervals up to months or years between time of administration of these modes. (6) Correction factors applied for radiation dose must take into account the maturation of each organ irradiated and not the child as a unit. The doses recommended for several organs appears to be in the same range as for adults: heart, kid-

Table IV. Dose recommendations in children and adults

		Children (CCSG)[1]		Adults TD$_{5/5}$[34]
Liver	whole	3,000 rad	4 weeks	2,500 rad
	partial	4,500 rad	5 weeks	4,500 rad
Lung	whole	1,800 rad	1½ weeks	1,500 rad
	partial	5,000 rad	5–6 weeks	4,000 rad
Heart	whole	1,800 rad	1½ weeks	4,000 rad
	partial	4,500 rad	5 weeks	5,500 rad
Kidney	whole	1,500–2,000 rad	4 weeks	2,000 rad
Brain	whole	4,500 rad	5 weeks	5,000 rad

[1] Children's cancer study group, Hepatoma III Study (CCG 881).

ney, lung, liver (table IV). Data available in the current literature suggest two periods of increased sensitivity: the first years of life, and the puberty growth spurt. This latter applies for the genital organs, bone and muscle.

References

1   Aronin, P.A.; Mahaley, M.S., Jr.; Rudnick, S.A.; Dudka, L.; Donohue, J.R.; Selker, R.G.; Moore, P.: Prediction of BCNU pulmonary toxicity in patients with malignant gliomas: an assessment of risk factors. new Engl. J. Med. *303:* 183–187 (1980).

2   Bleyer, W.A.; Griffin, T.W.: White matter necrosis, mineralizing microangiopathy and intellectual abilities in survivors of childhood leukemia: associations with central nervous system irradiation and methotrexate therapy in radiation damage to the nervous system; in Gilbert Kagan, pp. 155–174 (Raven Press, New York 1980).

3   Bloom, H.J.G.: Concepts in the natural history and treatment of medulloblastoma in children: increasing survival rates and possible risks with current radiotherapy techniques. CRC crit. Rev. radiol. Sci. *2:* 89 (1971).

4   Brasel, J.A.; Gruen, R.K.: Cellular growth: Brain, liver, muscle and lung; in Falkner, Tanner, Human growth, vol. 2, Potential growth, pp. 3–19 (Plenum Press, New York 1978).

5   Brodie, A.G.: Late growth changes in the human face. Angle Orthod. *23:* 146–157 (1953).

6   Carmel, R.J.; Kaplan, H.S.: Mantle irradiation in Hodgkin's disease: an analysis of technique, tumor irradication and complications. Cancer *37:* 2813–2825 (1976).

7   Castellino, R.A.; Glatstein, E.; Turbow, M.M.; Rosenberg, S.; Kaplan, H.S.: Latent radiation injury of lungs or heart activated by steroid withdrawal. Ann. Med., Hagerstown *80:* 593–599 (1976).

8 Chan, P.Y.M.; Kagan, A.R.; Byfield, J.E.; Rao, A.A.; Gilbert, H.A.; Nussbaum, H.: Pulmonary complications of combined chemotherapy and radiotherapy in lung cancer; in Vaeth Front. Radiat. Ther. Onc., vol 13, pp. 136–144 (Karger, Basel 1979).

9 Clemente, C.D.; Yamazaki, J.N.; Bennett, L.R.; McFall, R.A.: Brain radiation in newborn rats and differential effects of increased age. II. Microscopic observations. Neurology *10:*669–675 (1960).

10 Crosley, C.J.; Rorke, L.B.; Evans, A.; Nigro, M.: Central nervous system lesions in childhood leukemia. Neurology *28:*678–685 (1978).

11 Dekaban, A.S.: Abnormalities in children exposed to x-radiation during various stages of gestation: tentative timetable of radiation to the human fetus. Part I. J. nucl. Med. *9:*471–477 (1968).

12 DeSmet, A.A.; Kuhns, L.R.; Fayos, J.V.; Holt, D.T.: Effects of radiation therapy on growing long bones. Am. J. Rad, *127:*935–940 (1976).

13 Dobbing, J.; Sands, J.: The quantitative growth and development of the human brain. Archs Dis. Childh. *48:*757–767 (1973).

14 Falkner, F.; Tanner, J.M.: Human growth, vol. 1–3 (Plenum Press, New York 1978/1979).

15 Fryer, C.J.H.; Fitzpatrick, P.J.; Rider, W.D.; Poon, P.: Radiation pneumonitis: experience following a large single dose of radiation. Int. J. Radiat. Oncol. Biol. Phys. *4:*931–936 (1978).

16 Hall, E.J.: Radiobiology for radiologists; 2nd ed. (Harper & Row, New York 1978).

17 Hodson, W.a.: Development of the lung (Dekker, New York 1977).

18 Johnston, F.E.: somatic growth of the infant and preschool child; in Falkner, Tanner, Human growth, vol. 2, Potential growth, pp. 91–116 (Plenum Press, New York 1978).

19 Kramer, S.; Southard, M.E.; Mansfield, C.M.: Radiation effects and tolerance of the central nervous system: in Vaeth, Front. Radiat. Ther. Onc. vol. 6, pp. 332 (Karger, Basel 1972).

20 Littman, P.; Meadows, A.T.; Polgar, G.; Borns, P.F.; Rubin, E.: Pulmonary function in survivors of Wilms's tumor: patterns of impairment. Cancer *37:*2773–2776 (1976).

21 Maroteaux, P.; Faure, C.; Fessard, C.; Rigault, P.: Bone diseases of children, pp. 3–30 (Lippincott Company, Philadelphia 1979).

22 McIntosh, S.; Klatskin, E.H.; O'Brien, R.T.; Aspnes, G.T.; Kammerer, B.L.; Snead, C.; Kalavsky, S.M.; Pearson, H.A.: Chronic neurologic disturbance in childhood leukemia. Cancer *37:*853–857 (1976).

23 Meadows, A.T.; Gordon, J.; Littman, P.; Fergusson, J.; Moss, K.: Changes in intellect and IQ following combined treatment to the brain. Conf. long term normal tissue effects of cancer treatment, Bethesda 1981.

24 Miller, R.W.: Delayed effects occurring within the first decade after exposure of young individuals to the Hiroshima atomic bomb. Pediatrics, Springfield *18:*1–18 (1956).

25 Neuhauser, E.B.; Wittenborg, M.H.; Berman, C.Z.; Cohen, J.: Irradiation effects of roentgen therapy on the growing spine. Radiology *59:*637–650 (1952).

26 Newton, K.A.; Spittle, M.F.: An analysis of 40 cases treated by total thoracic irradiation. Clin. Radiol. *20:*19–22 (1969).

27 Parker, B.P.: Late effects of therapeutic irradiation on the skeleton and bone marrow. Cancer *37:*1162–1171 (1976).

28 Penney, D.P.; Rubin, P.: Specific early fine structural changes in lung following irradiation. Int. J. Radat. Oncol. Biol. Phys. *2:*1123–1132 (1977).

29 Penney, D.P.; Shapiro, D.L.; Rubin, P.; Finkelstein, J.: Long-term effects of radiation on the mouse lung and potential induction of radiation pneumonitis. Int. J. Radiat. Oncol. Biol. Phys. (to be published).

30 Price, R.A.; Birdwell, D.A.: the central nervous system in childhood leukemia. III. Mineralizing microangiopathy and dystrophic calcification. Cancer *42:* 717–728 (1978).

31 Price, R.A.; Jamieson, P.A.: The central nervous system in childhood leukemia. II. Subacute leukoencephalopathy. Cancer *35:*306–318 (1975).

32 Probert, J.C.; Parker, B.P.: The effects of radiation therapy on bone growth. Radiology *114:*155–162 (1975).

33 Rabinowicz, T.: The differentiated maturation of the human cortex. Neurol. Nutr. *3:*97–123 (1979).

34 Rubin, P.; Casarett, G.W.: Clinical radiation pathology, vol I, II (Saunders, Philadelphia 1968).

35 Rubin, P.: Dynamic classification of bone dysplasias (Year Book Medical Publishers, Chicago, 1969).

36 Rugh, R.: The impact of ionizing radiation on the embryo and fetus. Am. J. Roentg. *89:*182–190 (1963).

37 Rugh, R.: Why radiology? Radiology *82:*917–920 (1964).

38 Russell, L.B.; Russell, W.L.: An analysis of the changing radiation response of the developing mouse embryo. J. cell. Physiol. *43:*(1954). suppl. 1, pp. 103–149.

39 Shalet, S.M.; Beardwell, C.G.; Pearson, D.; Jones, P.H.M.: The effect of varying doses of cerebral irradiation on growth hormone producton in childhood. Clinical Endocr. *5:*287–290 (1976).

40 Silverman, C.L.; Thomas, P.R.; McAlister, W.H.; Walker, S.; Whiteside, L.A.: Slipped femoral capital epiphyses in irradiated children: dose volume and age relationships. Int. J. Radiat. Oncol. biol. Phys. (in press).

41 Simon, G.; Reiol, L.; Tanner, S.M.; Goldstein, H.; Benjamin, B.: Growth of radiobiologically determined heart diameter, lung width and lung lengths from 5–19 years with standard for clinical use. Archs. Dis. Childh. *47:*373–382 (1972).

42 Tanner, J.M.: Growth at adolescense (Blackwell Scientific Publications, Oxford 1962).

43 Tanner, J.M.; Whitehouse, R.H.; Takaishi, M.: Standard from birth to maturity for height, weight, height velocity and weight velocity. British children 1965. Archs. Dis. Childh. *41:*454–471 (1966).

44 Tanner, J.M.: Physical growth and development; in Forfar, Arneil, Textbook of Pediatrics, pp. 249–304 (Churvhill Livingston, Edingurgh 1978).

45 Tefft, M.: Radiation effect on growing bone and cartilage; in Vaeth. Front. Radiat. Ther. Onc., vol. 6, pp. 289–311 (Karger, Basel 1972).

46 Thurlbeck, W.M.: Postnatal growth and development of the lung. Am. Rev. resp. Dis. *111:*803–843 (1975).

47 Vaeth, J.M. (ed.): Combined effects of chemotherapy and radiotherapy on normal tissue tolerance. Front. Radiat. Ther. Onc. vol. 13 (Karger, Basel 1979).

48	Wara, W.M.; Phillips, T.L.; Margolis, L.W.; Smith, V.: radiation pneumonitis: a new approach to the derivation of time-dose factors. Cancer *32:* 547–552 (1973).

49	Weiss, B.R.; Muggia, F.M.: Cytotoxic drug-induced pulmonary disease: update 1980. Am. J. Med. *68:* 259–266 (1980).

50	Wohl, M.E.; Griscom, N.T.; Traggis, D.G.; Jaffe, N.: Effects of therapeutic irradiation delivered in early childhood upon subsequent lung function. Pediatrics, Springfield *55:* 507–516 (1975).

51	Yakovlev, P.I.; Lecours, A.R.; Minkowski, A.: Regional development of the brain in early life (Blackwell Scientific Publications, Oxford, 1967).

52	Yamazaki, J.N.; Bennett, L.R.; McFall, R.A.; Clemente, C.D.: Brain radiation in newborn rats and differential effects of increased age. I. Clinical observations. Neurology *10:* 530–536 (1960).

P. Rubin, MD, Division of Radiation Oncology, University of Rochester Medical Center, Rochester, NY 14627 (USA)

Front. Radiat. Ther. Onc., vol. 16, pp. 83–85 (Karger, Basel 1982)

Discussion

David: Dr. *Glaubiger,* what is the time period between phase I, phase II and phase III trials? It seems like a lot of the chronic side effects are not being picked up in the earlier trials.

Glaubiger: You mean in the animal trials?

David: Yes, and also in phase II and phase III. Are some of these chronic side effects being seen in some of the studies during phase II, animal studies?

Glaubiger: Some are, some are not. Cardiomyopathy, for example, is generally picked up in an animal study. With respect to your first question, phase II trials are normally not initiated until the phase I trial is completed. In other words, you have to have a maximum tolerated dose. As Dr. *Bleyer* pointed out, the phase I trials normally do not look for side effects that require months to years to appear, so a lot of the central nervous system toxicity that he was referring to would not be picked up by any current toxicity screen that is being used. Phase III trials, likewise, do not normally begin until phase II trials are completed. I do not know of any cases where drugs have been put in combination prior to being tested against specific tumors.

David: Chronic side effects occur from previous treatment. Looking to the future, how do Dr. *Bleyer* and Dr. *Rubin* anticipate cutting down on some of these chronic side effects? Would you look to cutting down on chemotherapy by the number of drugs given, the doses given? Should radiation doses be decreased or cut out altogether as in some of the trials? What is the best way we can look to the future of having some of these chronic side effects cut down by the combination of both treatments?

Bleyer: From a chemotherapy perspective there is not going to be a single way, it is going to be a multidisciplined attempt. Phase I, phase II trials, indeed, include agents that are thought to be less toxic, for example, the antracycline derivatives that are coming along look to be less cardiomyopathic-inducing. In the clinic, learning how to use old drugs in a safer way, better dosage schedules, is another point of attack. Learning how to combine drugs with the other therapeutic modalities, e.g. radiation, is important. To be very specific for a moment, since I mentioned brain dysfunction as one of the more common problems in children with leukemia, perhaps giving methotrexate before irradiation, a sequence in which irradiation is offered after methotrexate declines from plasma and spinal fluid is going to be less toxic than concurrent or the reverse order. As a single answer, there are many ways which are being attempted and in the future which will continue to be attempted.

Rubin: I think one of the big problems is that there is not any really good late effects program going on at NCI right now. The whole drug program has been an acute effect program to get drugs out, and one of the problems we have to get into, as I indicated, is the modeling. We cannot blanket areas. I think the idea of sequencing the modes is very important. There may be some real advantages for chemotherapy going first. We see this in the hematopoietic area where it could be that the utilization of these agents may actually be radioprotective. We might even be able to get a better response after we irradiate. We do not really understand what the basic units are. I think we are going to find there are some critical periods where that child is very vulnerable. If you begin going with all the modes at that time, there is no question that there is going to be a price tag on it. It is important to have a historical perspective. Those of us who began in radiation therapy also thought we would have minimum side effects. You need to be a long-term survivor to get a complication. But I think we clearly need the biological systems now to begin looking at late effects. In the combined modality era there is no question it is very critical.

Jaffe: I would like to congratulate the speakers on very fine presentations, and perhaps I can just offer a few comments. In analyzing the various data, one should also take into consideration race. For example, I have found that black people are able to tolerate doses of methotrexate far greater than white individuals. There is a tremendous excretion in the kidneys as far as the black person is concerned. I think this could also apply to some of the data that Dr. *Glaubiger* presented. There was no mention made of the various tolerances by the different races in regard to chemotherapy. There are differences in response of the adult vs. the child. Dr. *Bleyer's* data on the delayed effects of offspring in patients who have received chemotherapy is identical to that which we published from the Sydney Farber Cancer Institute about 3 years ago. It indicates that once a patient becomes pregnant, or once an individual can father a child, the offspring apparently does not have any delayed effects attributable to chemotherapy. What this will do in the future generation remains to be determined. One should not be very complacent about the possibility of chemotherapeutic agents causing second malignant neoplasms, but I am concerned about the alkylating agents. More and more data is being accumulated now in the adult that alkylating agents have been causing different types of neoplasms. This may certainly occur in children. Finally, with respect to some of the remarks made by Dr. *Rubin,* I will point out that the radiation delivered to a bone may not cause an immediate complication, and, in fact, one may never see a complication, but it does render the bone somewhat more susceptible to other side effects. For example, I recently analyzed the incidence of radiation-induced osteochondromas at the M.D. Anderson Hospital and Tumor Institute in pediatric patients. The incidence was 6% and then in analyzing the data further, I found that 2 or 3 of the patients had been subjected to some trauma at the sites. Had I ignored the trauma, the radiation-induced osteochondroma would have been approximately 4%.

D'Angio: If I could just make three quick comments on Dr. *Rubin's* presentation to emphasize some of the points that he was making. First, needless to say, it is a very complicated issue, but insofar as the immediate effects of irradiating, let us say growing bone, that may not be evident, it is rather parallel to what Dr. *Jaffe* just said. One does not see some of the effects until there is a call to proliferation. Very often in a growing bone, for example, the spine in Wilms' tumor patients, nothing is seen until the real spurt of adolescence, and then the changes are seen. The time to assess late effects is an important issue. The second point is the problems with animal models. The newborn rat is not the equivalent of the newborn human. If one uses the eye-opening reflex as more or less the equivalent age, then the newborn rat is no more, or rather the 17-day-old rat is no more sensitive to radiation therapy than, let us say, a 30-day-old rat. One has to be very careful about the models that are used insofar as these kinds of analyses are concerned. Third, insofar as applying any blanket formula, I could not agree more with Dr. *Rubin,* the dose adjustment that was used in Wilms' tumor applied only to flank irradiation. In the National Wilms' Tumor Study, for example, there is no dose adjustment with respect to the tolerance of the lung, and each tissue has to be considered separately.

David: Do you think there is a dose adjustment with regard to the tumor? Do you think the tumor changes in sensitivity at all?

D'Angio: No, that was never implied by that dose adjustment. It really was what the traffic would bear. I do not think the tumor cell knows how old it is.

Front. Radiat. Ther. Onc., vol. 16, pp. 86–89 (Karger, Basel 1982)

Bone Marrow Transplants

F. Leonard Johnson

Department of Hematology/Oncology, Children's Orthopedic Hospital and
Medical Center, Seattle, Wash., USA

Three major advances during the decade of the 1960s have enabled
marrow transplantation following high dose cytotoxic therapy to be
again considered as a means of treating childhood leukemia: definition
of the major histocompatibility complex (MHC) in man, development
of effective immunosuppressive agents, and improvements in supportive care with platelet and granulocyte transfusions, broad spectrum
antibiotics and hyperalimentation.

Initially, transplants for leukemia were performed in patients
refractory to chemotherapy with no expectation of further disease-free
survival. Several preparative regimens were used to eradicate the leukemia and allow engraftment, but the majority of these studies had
similar long-term survival rates of only 10% [4]. The medial survival of
the first 52 children transplanted for acute leukemia in the Seattle series
was 3 months [14] and 7 currently remain in remission from 5 to 9 years
following transplantation. These transplants failed because of graft
versus host disease (GVHD) in 17 patients (33%), relapse in 15 (29%),
and opportunistic infection in 5 (10%). 2 patients died, and 3 are living
with chronic GVHD.

Many of these patients died because of their poor clinical condition at the time of transplantation, and so in the second half of the
1970s marrow transplantation was performed earlier in the course of
leukemia, in acute lymphoblastic leukemia (ALL) during a second or
subsequent remission and in acute nonlymphoblastic leukemia (ANL)
after a first remission had been obtained. Results from three centers
have now shown that earlier transplantation markedly reduces the high
early mortality and morbidity of the procedure and enables 40–60% of
the patients to obtain long-term remissions [2, 11, 15, 16]. The com-

bined published results of the three largest series of children transplanted for ANL show that 13 of 16 remain in remission from 7 to 31 months, 2 having chronic GVHD [2, 11, 15]. 1 patient relapsed at 20 months and 2 died of severe GVHD. 9 of 19 children transplanted for ALL in a second or subsequent remission remain in continuing complete remission from 15 to 31 months [16]. The major cause of failure was relapse in 8 patients (42%).

Encouraging as these early results are, many challenges remain. Relapse still occurs in approximately half the remission transplants for ALL. Particularly disturbing is the observation of relapses as late as 39 months following remission transplantation for ALL when the patient's preparation included cyclophosphamide and total body irradiation [6], and 5½ years for ANL when the patient was transplanted in relapse following combination chemotherapy [9].

The incidence of fatal acute GVHD appears to be less in patients transplanted in remission, although the reason for this is unknown [2, 11, 15, 16]. Controlled studies have shown that prednisone is as effective a treatment as antithymocyte globulin (ATG) [17]. More recently, cyclosporin A has been investigated as a means of preventing GVHD, though its toxicity may be a limiting factor in its use [10]. If the abnormalities of T cell populations underlying both acute and chronic GVHD can be defined, the specific methods for prevention or therapy may not be long in development [12].

Chronic GVHD produces debilitating medical problems in a patient otherwise free of leukemia. The use of prednisone and azothioprine has improved the condition in some patients [13].

Treatment with marrow transplantation is available to a limited number of patients if donors are restricted to siblings completely matched at the A, B and D loci of the MHC. Successful transplants for leukemia have now been reported, however, where the donor was not a complete A, B and D match [3], or was unrelated but matched at the A, B and D loci [5], introducing the feasibility of banks of potential marrow donors. With the development of specific monoclonal antibodies against leukemia antigens, it may be possible to develop a leuke mia-free autologous marrow preparation for reinfusion. There is data in 1 patient that such a marrow will graft [7], but no data on how therapeutic this approach will be.

The most recent problem to be encountered following transplantation is leukoencephalopathy. In a large serie sof patients transplanted for ALL in relapse, approximately 25% had evidence of relapse in the central nervous system (CNS) [14], but no patient developed leukoencephalopathy. To reduce this incidence of CNS relapse, intrathecal methotrexate was added post-transplant [16] and several patients have now developed necrotising leukoencephalopathy, in one series 4 of 24 children transplanted for ALL in remission [6].

The most intriguing observation from this past decade of transplantation is that GVHD may play a role in the prevention of leukemic recurrence. The antileukemic effect of GVHD in leukemic models in rodents has been known since 1957 when it was demonstrated that allogeneic transplants produced fatal GVHD, but such afflicted animals were free of leukemia [1]. A similar association in humans has recently been reported [8, 18]. Relapse in patients who recovered from moderate to severe GVHD was 2½ times less than in patients who developed no, or minimal, GVHD [18]. This is of immense biological significance in our understanding of immunity and cancer, but presents a practical dilemma while we are currently unable to control GVHD.

Despite these current problems, marrow transplantation following high dose chemotherapy and radiation therapy has been the one new therapy introduced in the past decade that has offered the chance of improving the prognosis of children with acute leukemia. The lessons learned from this past decade in acute leukemia may also find application in other forms of childhood cancer such as non-Hodgkin's lymphoma, neuroblastoma, metastatic rhabdomyosarcoma and Ewing's sarcoma where chemotherapy and radiation produce definite, but usually transient, responses.

With the acceleration in our understanding and utilization of marrow transplantation over the past 10 years the decade of the 1980s holds exciting potential for marrow transplantation in the treatment of childhood cancer.

References

1   Berner, D.W.H.; Loutit, J.F.: Treatment of murine leukemia with X-rays and homologous bone marrow. Br. J. Hematol. *3:* 241–252 (1957).
2   Blume, K.G.; Beutler, E.; Bross, K.J.; et al.: Bone-marrow ablation and allogeneic marrow transplantation in acute leukemia. New Engl. J. Med *302:* 1041–1046 (1980).

3   Clift, R.A.; Hansen, J.S.; Thomas, E.D.; et al.: Marrow transplantation for donors other than HLA identical siblings. Transplantation *28:*235–424 (1979).

4   Gale, R.P.: Current status of bone marrow transplantation in acute leukemia. Transplant. Proc. *11:*1920–1923 (1979).

5   Hansen, J.A.; Clift, R.; Thomas, E.D.; et al.: Transplantation of marrow from an unrelated donor to a patient with acute leukemia. New Engl. J. Med. *305:*565–567 (1980).

6   Johnson, F.L.; Thomas, E.D.; Clark, B.; et al.: A comparison of marrow transplantation to chemotherapy for children with acute lymphoblastic leukemia in second or subsequent remission (submitted).

7   Netzel, B.; Haas, R.J.; Rodt, H.; et al.: Immunological conditioning of bone marrow for autotransplantation in childhood acute lymphoblastic leukemia. Lancet *i:* 1330–1332 (1980).

8   Odom, L.E.; August, C.S.; Githens, J.H.; et al.: Remission of relapsed leukemia during graft-versus-host reaction. A 'graft-versus-host leukemia reaction' in man? Lancet *ii:*537–540 (1978).

9   Oliff, R.; Ramu, N.P.; Poplack, D.: Leukemia relapse 5½ years after allogeneic bone marrow transplantation. Blood *52:*281–284 (1978).

10   Powles, R.L.; Clink, H.M.; Spence, D.; et al.: Cyclosporin – A to prevent graft-versus-host disease in man after allogeneic bone marrow transplantation. Lancet *i:* 327–329, (1980).

11   Powles, R.L.; Morgenstern, G.; Clink, H.M.; et al.: The place of bone marrow transplantation in acute myelogenous leukaemia. lancet *i:* 1047–1050 (1980).

12   Reinherz, E.L.; Parkman, R.; Rappaport, J.; et al.: Aberrations of suppressor T cells in human graft-versus host disease. New Engl. J. Med. *300:*1062–1068 (1979).

13   Sullivan, K.M.; Shulman, H.M.; Storb, R.; et al.: Chronic graft-versus-host disease in fifty-two patients. Adverse natural course and successful treatment with combination immunosuppression. Blood (in press).

14   Thomas, E.D.; Buckner, C.D.; Benaji, N.: One hundred patients with acute leukemia treated by chemotherapy, total body irradiation and allogeneic marrow transplantation. Blood *49:*511–533 (1977).

15   Thomas, E.D.; Buckner, C.D.; Clift, R.A.; et al.: Marrow transplantation for acute nonlymphoblastic leukemia in first remission. New Engl. J. Med. *301:* 597–599 (1979).

16   Thomas, E.D.; Sanders, J.E.; Flournoy, N.; et al.: Marrow transplantation for patients with acute lymphoblastic leukemia in remission. Blood *54:*468–476 (1979).

17   Weiden, P.L.; Doney, K.; Storb, R.; Thomas, E.D.: Antihyman thymocyte globulin (ATG for prophylaxis and treatment of graft-versus-host disease in recipients of allogeneic marrow grafts. Transplant. Proc. *10:*213–216 (1978).

18   Weiden, P.L.; Flournoy, N.; Thomas, E.D.; et al.: Antileukemic effect of graft-versus-host disease in human recipients of allogeneic marrow grafts. New Engl. J. Med. *300:*1068–1073 (1979).

F.L. Johnson, MD, Department of Hematology/Oncology,
St. Jude Children's Research Hospital, Memphis, TN 38101 (USA)

Front. Radiat. Ther. Onc., vol. 16, pp. 90–104 (Karger, Basel 1982)

Brain Gliomas in Children: Treatment Policy and Prognosis

H.J.G. Bloom[1]

Department of Radiotherapy, Royal Marsden Hospital and Institute of Cancer Research, London, England

Incidence and Mortality

In children the most common malignant tumours after leukaemia occur in the brain. For every 1 million children under age 15 in Britain and in the United States there are, each year, about 100 new cases of cancer [Epidemiology and End Results Programme, 1973–1976; *Birch* et al., 1980] of which approximately 20 will have tumours of the central nervous system. Among the children of England and Wales under age 15 we can expect annually approximately 200 new cases of brain tumour and 150 deaths from this cause. The corresponding figures in the United States are about 1,000 new cases and 750 deaths. In both these countries accidents still continue to take a greater toll of children's lives than all cancers put together; but what brain tumours may lack in actual numbers they make up for in the magnitude of disturbance caused to patient, family and medical staff, at the time of investigation and treatment, and often over many years to come, during which continued medical, social and educational supervision are required.

Tumour Types

The peak incidence of intracranial tumours in childhood occurs in the second half of the first decade. Just over half of all tumours develop

---

[1] I am grateful to Mr. *R. Skeet,* Director of the South Thames Cancer Registry for figures 1 and 2.

in the infratentorial region, the majority of which are astrocytomas of the cerebellum and brain stem, medulloblastomas and fourth ventricle ependymomas. Nearly 50% of tumours are found in the supratentorial region and consist principally of astrocytomas of the cerebral lobes, hypothalamus and optic chiasma, ependymomas of the third and lateral ventricles, craniopharyngiomas and pineal tumours. Per unit volume, more tumours in children occur in the posterior fossa and in relation to the third ventricle than in the much larger volume of the cerebral hemispheres which is by far the major site for brain tumours in adults.

Treatment

Brain gliomas, even of high grade malignancy, very rarely metastasize outside the cerebrospinal axis. They kill by raised intracranial pressure and by local effects. Therapeutic efforts against such lesions are therefore directed essentially towards controlling disease at the primary site. Some gliomas, especially medulloblastomas, and to a lesser extent ependymomas and germinomas, may spread via the CSF to other parts of the neuraxis. This is a significant complication but, unlike blood-borne metastases, eradication of CSF seedlings by treatment during the clinically occult stage often seems possible.

Surgery

Advances in surgical techniques, anaesthesia and supportive care have undoubtedly made operations for intracranial tumours safer. Even so, the risk to life and especially to cerebral function imposes a strict limitation on any radical surgical approach to gliomas. Nevertheless, surgery continues to play an important role in the management of these tumours by reducing intracranial pressure, thereby averting early death and preserving vision, by obtaining a tissue diagnosis and by debulking as much of the tumour as is safely possible. In this way surgery prepares the way for further treatment aimed at residual tumour.

Radiotherapy

Survival in patients with gliomas is increased by post-operative radiotherapy compared with surgery alone and this has been, and still remains, the most effective adjuvant treatment to date. Furthermore, in

those patients with deep-seated gliomas such as in the thalamus, hypothalamus or brain stem where surgery, even biopsy, is hazardous, radiotherapy alone reduces neurological disability in a high proportion of
cases and often prolongs useful life, sometimes for several or more
years. On the other hand, radiotherapy also has serious restrictions: the
extent to which the dose of irradiation can be increased is limited by
the risk to normal brain tissue, especially the developing central nervous system in young children.

We have recently reached what is virtually a surgical and radiothe-
rapeutic impasse in the treatment of intracranial tumours and efforts
are now being made to rise above this therapeutic plateau by the introduction of further adjuvants, principally chemotherapy and chemical
radiosensitizers.

Cytotoxic and Radiosensitizing Agents

Chemotherapy for brain tumours is directed, not at systemic disease, as with most other types of childhood malignancy, but towards
destroying the primary tumour and possible seedlings within the CSF
pathways. Chemotherapy for cerebral tumours is restricted by the
'blood-brain barrier' and the number of effective agents with the requi-
site chemico-physical properties to overcome this barrier is limited.
The principal agents in use at present against gliomas are the nitrosou-
reas, procarbazine and vincristine. Other cytotoxic compounds under
current study include VM_{26}, VP_{16}, methotrexate, dibromodulcitol, and
most recently, cis-platinum [*Klan* et al., 1980].

The most hopeful research at present in radiotherapy concerns
chemical agents which have a selective radiosensitizing action on radio-
resistent hypoxic tumour cells [*Adams* et al., 1980]. Current interest is
focussed on derivatives of nitroimidazole, principally misonidazole
[*Dische* et al., 1979; *Wasserman* et al., 1981]. These compounds are
remarkable in possessing both selective radiosensitizing and cytotoxic
properties against hypoxic tumour cells, with little or no action on normal well-oxygenated tissue.

General Prognosis

The outlook for children with brain gliomas is in general better
than for adults. This is largely but not entirely due to the preponder-

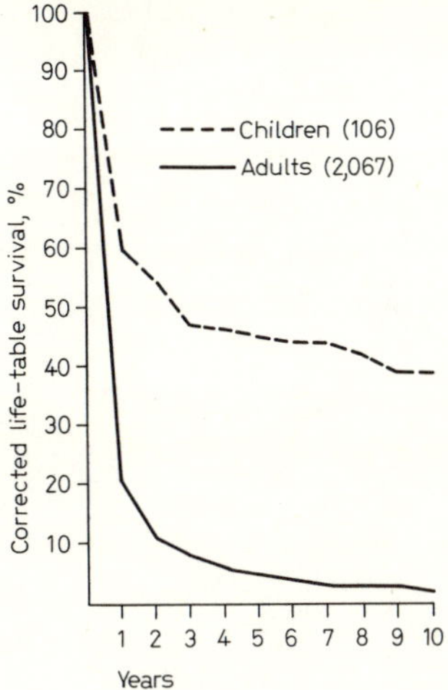

Fig. 1. Survival of all adults and children (age under 15) with histologically verified cerebral astrocytomas (all grades) registered within the region of South-East England covered by the South Thames Cancer Registry, 1958–1974.

ance of lower grade astrocytomas in children. At the South Thames Cancer Registry, covering a total population of some 6 million people in our geographical region, the survival rate for all children under age 15 registered with brain gliomas was substantially greater than for adults. This applied to astrocytomas of all grades, and also to unverified gliomas (fig. 1, 2). On the other hand, the prognosis for medulloblastoma and ependymoma was better in adults than in children [*Skeet,* pers. commun.].

I will refer to cerebral gliomas, since these tumours represent primary brain cancers and constitute some 80% of all intracranial tumours in children. I intend to draw mainly from experience at the Royal Marsden Hospital where between 1952 and 1976 a total of 461 new patients under age 16 with various types of intracranial tumour were referred for radiotherapy: 378 of these children had gliomas (82%). The overall 5- and 10-year survival rates for the entire series were 48 and 41%, respectively (fig. 3), the older children faring better than the young ones (fig. 4).

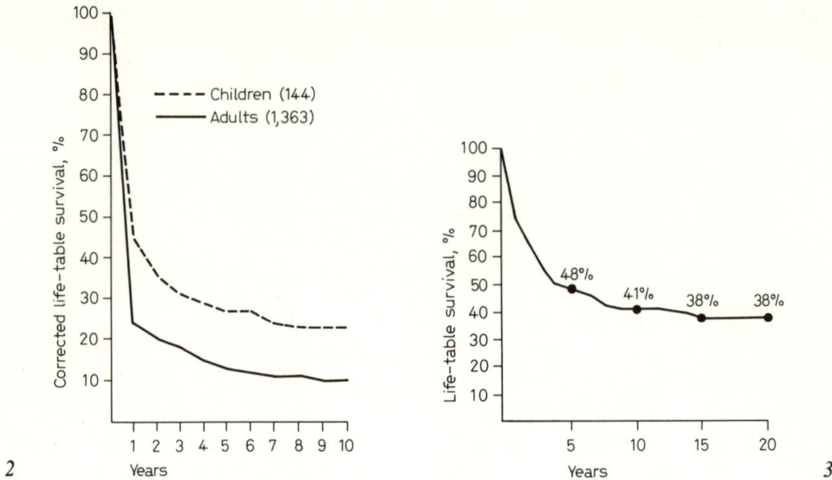

Fig. 2. As for figure 1, but concerned with histologically unverified cerebral tumours.

Fig. 3. Survival of all chidren (n = 461), age 15 years or less, with all types of primary intracranial tumour referred to the Royal Marsden for radiotherapy, 1952–1976.

Tumours of the Cerebral Hemispheres

About 25% of intracranial tumours in children are located in the cerebral hemispheres. The majority are astrocytomas of low or intermediate grade malignancy. When surgery is feasible, as much of the neoplasm as possible is removed and this should be followed by large volume radical radiotherapy. Many tumours, however, are deep-seated and inoperable, such as those occurring in the thalamus, hypothalamus and around the walls of the 3rd ventricle. These cases are treated by radiotherapy alone, with or without a preliminary CSF shunt.

Because of their well-differentiated histology and often slow growth, low grade astrocytomas are often regarded as being resistant to radiotherapy. The available evidence suggests that this is not the case and that such tumours do respond to irradiation, leading to greater post-operative survival than following surgery alone [*Bouchard,* 1966; *Bloom and Walsh,* 1975; *Leibel* et al., 1975; *Fazekas,* 1977].

Fortunately, the dreaded high grade astrocytoma or glioblastoma is uncommon in children. Under age 16 this tumour constitutes only

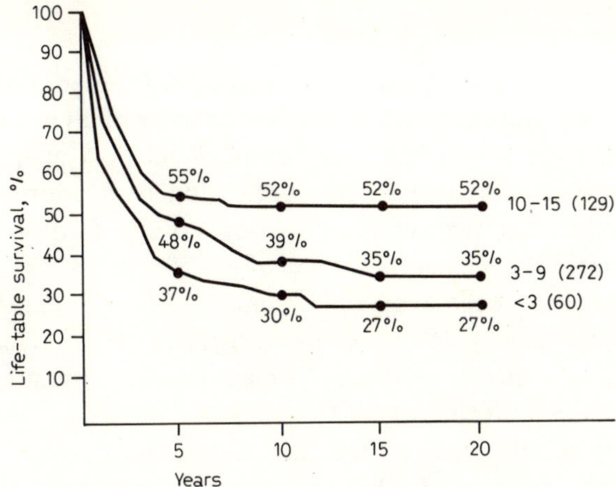

Fig. 4. Survival of all children (n = 461) with primary intracranial tumours referred to the Royal Marsden, 1952–1976, for radiotherapy according to three age categories.

Table I. Royal Marsden Hospital (1952–1976): cerebral hemisphere gliomas in children survival in all children (n = 122) referred for radiotherapy

Site	Patients	Survival[1], %		
		5 years	10 years	15 years
Cerebral lobes and lateral ventricles	59	46	39	39
3rd ventricle and hypothalamus	45	71	58	58
Thalamus	18	20	20	20

[1] 5-, 10- and 15-year survival rates for children with cerebral hemisphere gliomas (histologically verified and unverified) according to principal site.

about 5% of all intracranial tumours and may carry a somewhat better prognosis than a tumour of apparently comparable grade in adults.

The 5- to 15-year survival rates for 122 children with cerebral hemisphere gliomas of all types, verified and unverified, referred to the Royal Marsden for radiotherapy, according to principal site, are shown in table I.

Medulloblastoma

Medulloblastoma is the most malignant and most frequent type of brain cancer found in children, constituting 20% or more of all intracranial tumours (29% in the Royal Marsden series). With post-operative radiotherapy to the whole neuraxis, the application of more precise megavoltage techniques and the use of higher doses of irradiation, particularly to the posterior fossa, survival rates of 30–50% at 5 years, and up to 30% at 10 years have been achieved [*Pearson*, 1974; *Bloom*, 1977, 1979a; *Harisiadis and Chang*, 1977; *Mealey and Hall*, 1977; *Schweisguth*, 1979]. This is in contrast to the 0–10% associated with surgery alone or with inadequte radiotherapy.

It is important to appreciate that the encouraging results for medulloblastoma from major radiotherapy centres are often based on selected cases with exclusion of patients dying before, during and soon after operation, and often of cases who fail to complete treatment.

Medulloblastoma is an undifferentiated embryonic tumour and one hoped that,like other such tumours in childhood, it would respond to chemotherapy. However, it was assumed that adjuvant chemotherapy in such cases could produce haematological problems during treatment due to depletion of marrow reserve by the combined effects of whole cerebrospinal axis irradiation and cytotoxic drugs. In 1970 a pilot study of such combined modality treatment was started at the Royal Marsden Hospital [*Bloom*, 1975]. We have treated a total of 37 children with adjuvant chemotherapy using vincristine during radiotherapy, followed by intermittent courses of CCNU and vincristine every 6 weeks over 12 months. Early in the study some patients received 4 courses of intrathecal methotrexate during or after the last 2 weeks of radiotherapy. This multimodal treatment proved feasible and apparently beneficial since survival was substantially greater than for a historical series of 88 patients from the same Centre in which chemotherapy was not used (fig. 5).

The encouraging early results of this pilot study led to a randomised multi-centre trial being set up in 1975 through the International Society of Paediatric Oncology (SIOP) to test the value of adjuvant chemotherapy for medulloblastoma and also high grade ependymoma. 44 centres from 15 countries entered 287 cases of medulloblastoma into the study which was closed at the end of 1979. The full treatment schedule has been reported elsewhere [*Bloom*, 1979a, b].

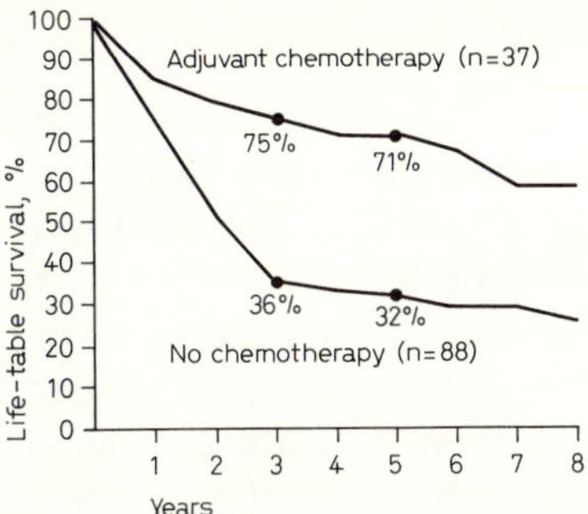

Fig. 5. Survival of children with medulloblastoma treated by surgery, post-operative cerebrospinal axis radiotherapy and adjuvant chemotherapy (principally vincristine and CCNU), 1970–1980. This is compared with 88 historical controls at the same centre (1952–1969) who did not receive chemotherapy.

Intermediate results were presented by the author on behalf of the Brain Tumour Committee to the SIOP Annual Conference in Budapest, September 1980. The disease-free actuarial survival of patients receiving adjuvant chemotherapy was better than for the non-chemotherapy group and the difference had reached a level of limited statistical significance (p = 0.029). At 3 years, 62% of 140 patients in the chemotherapy arm were alive and disease-free, compared with 49% of 140 in the non-chemotherapy arm. Various subsets showed a survival trend, often not significant, in favour of the adjuvant chemotherapy. These results from a controlled multicentre trial together with those from the non-controlled Royal Marsden Hospital study (fig. 5) suggest that chemotherapy could come to play an important role in the multimodal management of medulloblastoma. More advanced results from the SIOP trial and from a similar study in the USA [*Evans* et al., 1979] are awaited. In the meantime, various paediatric-oncologic groups are examining new and hopefully more effective cytotoxic drug regimens, including so-called 'sandwich' chemotherapy which is administered during the interval between surgery and radiotherapy: high dose methotrexate with citrovorum factor rescue, alone or in combination with other drugs, is being used for this purpose [*Voûte,* 1980; *Neidhardt and Reihm,* 1980, pers. commun.).

Cerebellar Astrocytomas

The cerebellar astrocytoma is one of the most important tumours met with in childhood since it constitutes approximately 20% of all intracranial tumours and frequently is amenable to total excision. In such circumstances the cure rate is expected to be 100%. However, there appear to be two distinct types of cerebellar astrocytoma based on histological criteria – the more frequent juvenile piloid lesion characterised by Rosenthal fibres and associated with a 25-year survival rate in excess of 90%, and a less common diffuse type of which only some 40% of patients are still alive at 25 years [*Gjerris and Klinken,* 1978]. In about 30% of all patients total tumour removal is not possible: in such cases post-operative irradiation appears useful [*Griffin* et al., 1979] and is recommended, especially for astrocytomas of the diffuse type or of higher grade and when there is invasion of the brain stem.

Results of treatment for cerebellar astrocytomas from radiotherapy departments obviously cannot be compared with purely neurosurgical series, since only the worse cases are referred for the ancillary treatment. Of a total of 30 children with unfavourable cerebellar astrocytomas referred to the Royal Marsden Hospital for post-operative radiotherapy, 70% were alive at 5 years and 58% at 10–20 years.

Brain Stem Tumours

True brain stem gliomas consist of intrinsic neoplasms of the medulla and pons and make up about 10% of all intracranial tumours in childhood. They cause considerable disability and distress from involvement of closely packed neurogenic components in a small vital anatomical structure which forms the highway for information between body and brain. In most patients the diagnosis is based on clinical and radiological features since surgery, even when limited to biopsy, is dangerous. There is a high initial response rate to radiotherapy with clinical improvement in 70–75% of cases [*Marsa* et al., 1973; *Sheline,* 1975]. Unfortunately, this early benefit is not maintained and recurrence, resulting in progressive disability and early death generally within 2 years, is the fate of the majority of patients. The overall 5-year survival rate is in the region of 15–20% and this has been our experience at the Royal Marsden Hospital and that of other centres [*Schweisguth,* 1979; *Hendrick* et al., 1975; *Marsa* et al., 1973].

Royal Marsden Hospital Series

57 children with tumours of the brain stem were referred for radiotherapy, 10 of whom failed to complete treatment. At 5 years only 17% of all cases were still alive, and this figure was maintained to 20 years. Therapeutic failure led to a rapidly fatal outcome: death occurred in 60% of the patients within 12 months.

Gliomas of the brain stem present a great challenge to the radiotherapist. They consist of relatively small and inoperable tumour burdens, show good initial responses to irradiation, but develop early local recurrence without dissemination in over 80% of cases. Clearly, the situation seems ideal for exploring the value of chemical radiosensitizers in the hope of rendering local residual hypoxic tumour tissue more vulnerable to treatment.

Royal Marsden Hospital Misonidazole Study

We are at present conducting a pilot study with misonidazole in the primary treatment of children with brain stem tumours. The sensitizer is given in daily oral doses of 600 mg/m^2 during the last 4 weeks of a 6-week course of radical megavoltage radiotherapy (total tumour dose 5,000 rad). It is administered 4 h prior to irradiation which produces blood levels of between 30 and 40 µg/ml. It is too early to refer to results but it can be said that misonidazole has been surprisingly well tolerated. This may be due to concomitant steroid administration which appears to reduce neurotoxicity, but which may also interfere with radiosensitization [*Bloom and Bugden*, 1981; *Walker and Strike*, 1980].

Ependymomas

Ependymomas arise from the lining of the ventricular system and constitute about 10% of all intracranial tumours in children with about 40% occurring above, and 60% below the tentorium. High dose, large volume post-operative radiotherapy is essential if the maximum cure rate is to be achieved [*Salazar* et al., 1975; *Bloom*, 1981].

Tumour seeding within the CSF pathways is a feature of ependymomas, occurring more frequently with posterior fossa tumours, especially when of high grade malignancy [*Bloom and Walsh*, 1975; *Kim and Fayos*, 1977; *Bloom*, 1981]. For all patients with high grade tumours and for all those with posterior fossa lesions we recommend extension of treatment to include the whole cerebrospinal axis. For patients with low grade supratentorial ependymomas treatment is limited to the primary region but with a generous margin of clearance.

Royal Marsden Hospital Series

Of 47 children with ependymoma referred for radiotherapy, 53% survived 5 years and 37% 10 years, with 32% still alive at 20 years.

Prognosis for ependymoma is largely dependent on the grade of malignancy: general experience shows that for grade I and II cases the 5-year survival rate is between 50 and 75%, compared with only 15–20% for those with grade III–IV lesions. Because of poor results in patients with high grade ependymomas following surgery and radiotherapy we carried out a pilot study with adjuvant chemotherapy at the Royal Marsden using the same programme as for medulloblastomas. Although the early results in a small series were encouraging (69% 5-year survival compared with 44% in historical controls) improvement with chemotherapy was not maintained beyond 6–7 years. In the SIOP trial, so far, there is no difference between the survival of children with high grade ependymomas receiving or not receiving adjuvant chemotherapy. These tumours obviously do not respond so well to chemotherapy as do medulloblastomas: a different type of cytotoxic drug combination may be more successful.

Late Effects

In no other condition can there be more concern over possible late sequelae and the subsequent quality of life as following the successful treatment of a child with a brain glioma, especially as survival rates for such patients seem to be increasing in recent years. In the Royal Marsden series the 5-year survival rate for children completing treatment for various gliomas by type or site ranges from as high as 78 down to 19%: the corresponding 10-year rates are 63 and 19%, respectively (fig. 6). In our total series of 461 children there were 60 who were treated under age 3, at a time when the developing central nervous system may be particularly vulnerable to the effects of disease and treatment. 30% of this youngest group were still alive at 10 years (fig. 4): the corresponding figure for those completing radiotherapy was 36%.

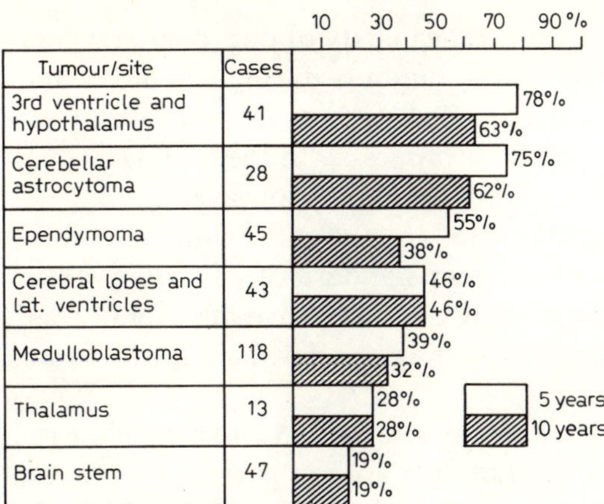

Fig. 6. Histogram showing 5- and 10-year survival rates by tumour type/site of 335 children of a total of 378 with cerebral gliomas who completed radical radiotherapy, post-operatively or alone, at the Royal Marsden Hospital, 1952–1976.

The dose/time factors generally employed in radiotherapy appear to be safe, as far as *gross* radiation damage to the brain is concerned. We are on less certain grounds in relation to the production of more subtle irradiation-induced tissue changes which may lead to neuropsychological disturbances and to hypothalamic-pituitary endocrine deficiency. Impaired intellect and learning ability following treatment of brain tumours, generally ascribed to irradiation, have been reported by *Bamford* et al. [1976] and by *Raimondi and Tomita* [1979]. On the other hand, several authors, have commented favourably on the overall functional results in children treated for brain tumours by irradiation, some 70–80% of all surviving cases apparently leading 'active useful' lives [*Bloom,* 1979b]. The criteria for this assessment has been crude and usually based on general clinical observation and social enquiry. Clearly, a more detailed and more precise assessment of intellectual capabilities and psychosocial relationships are needed by specially trained personnel. The effects of irradiation on the brain depend upon the dose per individual fraction, the total dose reached and the overall time in which it is given. In any study on the subject these factors must be stated and correlated with end results and sequelae.

We are examining the mental capacity of our long-term survivors who were treated for intracranial tumours during childhood and who were alive and available for detailed study 4–18 years after treatment [*Eiser, Jannoun, Bloom,* study in progress]. In the first 47 patients the IQ scores were found to be within the high to low average range in 68% of cases and borderline in 13%. So far, 20% of the children in this preliminary study had reached a higher standard of education which suggests that perhaps more can be done to improve the overall results by proper counselling and by providing special facilities for 'catch-up' training.

It must be appreciated that any intellectual and behaviour changes in children treated for brain tumours are not necessarily the result of radiotherapy and chemotherapy. It is important to take into account the effects of the tumour itself, especially raised intracranial pressure. *Fischer* et al. [1968] performed neuropsychiatric and psychometric tests on 46 patients of varying age with brain tumours, on average 4.4 years after surgery *without* radiotherapy, and found examples of significant mental change, such as reduction of intellectual capacity, slowing of thought processes, changes in mood and limited self-control under stress.

Until we have found more efficient and more selective treatments for brain tumours we have to face accepting a possible reduction in mental capacity, perhaps some emotional disability and some neurogenic and endocrine dysfunction as the cost for an otherwise healthy and active child who will eventually be able to earn his own living, although perhaps at a reduced level. The effects of therapeutic irradiation on normal brain and other tissues have been considered in some detail elsewhere [*Bloom,* 1971].

A difficult situation may arise when the child with a brain tumour recovers or improves with treatment, returns to an active life but his family and teachers expect him to die soon.Plans for the child's future are suspended. Parents and relatives wait for the end. Educational efforts are half-hearted and considered to be a waste of time. There is disruption in the home and sometimes parents may quarrel and even part. For some children long-term survival brings its own special problems and in these circumstances we must strive to prevent therapeutic triumph being overshadowed by tragedy in the home and failure at school.

References

Adams, G.E.; Ahmed, I.; Fielden, E.M.; O'Neill, P.; Stratford, I.J.: The development of some nitroimidazoles as hypoxic cell sensitizers. Cancer clin. Trials *3:* 37–42 (1980).

Bamford, F.N.; Jones, P.M.; Pearson, D.; Ribeiro, G.G.; Shalet, S.M. Beardwell, C.G.: Residual disabilities in children treated for intracranial space-occupying lesions. Cancer *37:* 1149–1151 (1976).

Birch, J.M.; Marsden, H.B.; Swindell, R.: Incidence of malignant disease in childhood: a 24-year review of the Manchester Tumour Data. Br. J. Cancer *42:* 215–223 (1980).

Bloom, H.J.G.: Concepts in the natural history and treatment of medulloblastoma in children: increasing survival rates and possible risks with current radiotherapy techniques. CRC crit. Rev. radiol. Sci. *2:* 89–143 (1971).

Bloom, H.J.G.: Combined modality therapy for intracranial tumours. Cancer *35:* 111–120 (1975).

Bloom, H.J.G.: Medulloblastoma: prognosis and prospects (editorial). Int. J. Radiat. Oncol. Biol. Phys. *2:* 1031–1033 (1977).

Bloom, H.J.G.: Adjuvant therapy for residual disease in children with medulloblastoma; in Bonadonna, Mathé, Salmon, Recent results in cancer research, vd. *68:* pp. 412–422 (Springer, Berlin 1979a).

Bloom, H.J.G.: Recent concepts in the conservative treatment of intracranial tumours in children. Acta neurochir. *50:* 103–116 (1979b).

Bloom, H.J.G.: Recent results and research in the treatment of intracranial gliomas; in Chang, Housepian, Tumours of the central nervous system: modern radiotherapy in multidisciplinary management (Masson, New York 1981).

Bloom, H.J.G.; Bugden, R.D.: Radiation and misonidazole in children with brain stem gliomas and supratentorial glioblastoma: a pilot study. 2nd Int. Meet. on Progress in Radio-Oncology, Baden 1981 (to be published, 1981).

Bloom, H.J.G.; Walsh, L.: Tumours of the central nervous system; in Bloom, Lemerle, Neidhardt, Voûte, Cancer in children – clinical management, pp. 93–119 (Springer, Berlin 1975).

Bouchard, J.: Radiation therapy of tumours and diseases of the nervous system (Kimpton, London 1966).

Dische, S.; Saunders, M.I.; Flockhart, I.R.; Lee, M.E.; Anderson, P.: Misonidazole – a drug for trial in radiotherapy and oncology. Int. J. Radiat. Oncol. Biol. Phys. *5:* 851–860 (1979).

Evans, A.E.; Anderson, J.; Jenkin, R.D.T.; Kramer, S.; Schoenfeld, D.; Wilson, C.: Adjuvant chemotherapy for medulloblastoma and ependymoma: in Paoletti, Walker, Butti, Knerich, Multidisciplinary aspects of brain tumour therapy, pp. 219–222 (Elsevier/North-Holland, Amsterdam 1979).

Fazekas, J.T.: Treatment of grades I and II brain astrocytomas: the role of radiotherapy. Int. J. Radiat. Oncol. Biol. Phys. *2:* 661–666 (1977).

Fischer, P.-A.; Schmidt, G.; Wanke, K.: Neurologische, psychiatrische und testpsychologische Befunde nach der Behandlung von hirneigenen Tumoren. Neurochirurgia *11:* 98–112 (1968).

Griffin, T.W.; Beaufait, D.; Blasko, J.C.: Cystic cerebellar astrocytomas in childhood. Cancer *44:* 276–280 (1979).

Gjerris, F.; Klinken, L.: Long-term prognosis in children with benign cerebellar astrocytoma. J. Neurosurg. *49:*179–184 (1978).

Harisiadis, L.; Chang, C.H.: Medulloblastoma in children: a correlation between staging and results of treatment. Int. J. Radiat. Oncol. Biol. Phys. *2:*833–841 (1977).

Hendrick, E.B.; Hoffman, H.J.; Humphreys, R.P.: Treatment of infratentorial gliomas in childhood; in Hekmatpanah, Gliomas: current concepts in biology, diagnosis and therapy, pp. 102–106 (Springer, Berlin 1975).

Kim, Y.H.; Fayos, J.V.: Intracranial ependymomas. Radiology *124:*805–808 (1977).

Klan, A.; McCullough, D.; Borts, F.; Sinks, L.F.: Update on use of cis-platinum in CNS malignancies. Abstr. Proc. AACR and ASCO, C283 (1980).

Leibel, S.A.; Sheline, G.E.; Wara, W.M.; Boldrey, E.B., Neilson, S.L.: The role of radiation therapy in the treatment of astrocytomas. Cancer *35:*1551–1557 (1975).

Marsa, G.W.; Probert, J.C.; Rubinstein, L.J.; Bagshaw, M.A.: Radiation therapy in the treatment of childhood gliomas. Cancer *32:*646–655 (1973).

Mealey, J.; Hall, P.V.: Medulloblastoma in children: survival and treatment. J. Neurosurg. *46:*56–64 (1977).

Pearson, D.: Tumours of the central nervous system; in Deeley, Modern radiotherapy and oncology: malignant diseases in children, pp. 98–119 (Butterworths, London 1974).

Raimondi, A.J.; Tomita, T.: The disadvantages of prophylactic whole CNS post-operative radiation therapy for medulloblastoma; in Paoletti, Walker, Butti, Knerich, Multidisciplinary aspects of brain tumour therapy, pp. 209–218 (Elsevier/North-Holland, Amsterdam 1979).

Salazar, O.M.; Rubin, P.; Bassano, D.; Marcial, V.A.: Improved survival of patients with intracranial ependymomas by irradiation - dose selection and field extension. Cancer *35:*1563–1574 (1975).

Schweisguth, O.: Tumeurs solides de l'enfant, pp. 191–208 (Flammarion, Paris 1979).

Sheline, G.E.: Radiation therapy of tumours of the central nervous system in childhood. Cancer *35:*957–964 (1975).

Surveillance, Epidemiology and End Results (SEER) Programme (1973–76). US Department of Health, National Cancer Institute, Washington (US Govt. Printing Office).

Walker, M.D.; Strike, T.A.: Misonidazole peripheral neuropathy: its relationship to plasma concentration and other drugs. Cancer clin. Trials *3:*105–109 (1980).

Wasserman, T.H.; Stetz, J.; Phillips, T.L.: Clinical trials of misonidazole in the United States. Cancer clin. Trials *4:*7–16 (1981).

H.J.G. Bloom, MD, Department of Radiotherapy, Royal Marsden Hospital and Institute of Cancer Research, London SW3 (England)

Front. Radiat. Ther. Onc., vol. 16, pp. 105–113 (Karger, Basel 1982)

Malignant Bone Tumors in Children
A Decade of Progress[1]

Norman Jaffe

Department of Pediatrics, M.D. Anderson Hospital and Tumor Institute, Houston, Tex., USA

Introduction

During the past decade, major advances have been forged in the diagnosis and treatment of malignant bone tumors in children. These encompass newer diagnostic techniques, advances in chemotherapy, improvements in radiation, new criteria to assess response and identification of prognostic variables. These have led to refinement in therapy, innovative approaches, and escalation in cure and survival. This communication will review these advances and their impact on current concepts in management.

Newer Diagnostic Techniques

High resolution bone scintigraphy is a sensitive tool for detecting bone pathology. This investigative strategy has been utilized to identify skeletal metastases prior to their appearance on conventional radiographs [30]. It is also used to identify skip metastases and plan the level of transmedullary amputation. The latter is performed 7 cm proximal to the margin of radionuclide activity and has virtually elimated stump recurrence [20].

Tomographic and xeroradiographic studies of the primary tumor are also employed. They have been successful in identifying cortical transgression, pathologic fractures and soft tissue masses with greater clarity. Computerized tomography is also used to demonstrate the

[1] Supported in part by grants CA-03713-24 and P5/p16.

axial extent of tumor and skip metastases [11]. Its ability to delineate extra-osseous extension of disease permits more precise planning of the radiation portals. It may also identify pulmonary metastases not visible on conventional radiographs.

Major advances have also been achieved in tumor angiography. Selective catheterization has been utilized to administer chemotherapy and enhance the tumoricidal effect of active agents [21]. Responses achieved by this means have improved the safety of surgical resection. Similarly, vascular occlusion and tumor infarction have been utilized for definitive treatment in giant cell tumors an as an alternative to surgery for inoperable lesions [45].

Advances in Treatment

Osteosarcoma

During the past decade, the following chemotherapeutic agents were found to be effective in osteosarcoma: (1) high dose methotrexate with citrovorum factor (Citrovorum factor rescue) (MTX-CF) [22]; (2) adriamycin (ADR) [8]; (3) cis-dichloro-diammine platinum-II (CDP) [33].

The application of these agents in patients with established disease yielded responses of 30–40%. This prompted their use as adjuvant therapy after primary definitive treatment. The tactic was based on the premise that pulmonary micrometastases are present in a majority of patients at the time of diagnosis. Improvement in survival, therefore, could only be anticipated by eliminating the invisible tumor burden. The strategy proved successful. The 3- to 5-year survival was escalated to 50–80% as opposed to 20% in historical controls [8, 14, 23, 38, 42].

Enthusiasm generated by the impact of chemotherapy was instrumental in investigating limb salvage with functional restoration as an alternative to amputation. In the initial studies, high dose methotrexate alone or in combination with radiation and other agents was employed. This produced tumor destruction varying from 50 to 100% in 41 of 61 cases (67%) [13, 25, 37]. More recently, CDP, administered via the intra-arterial route to achieve greater tumoricidal concentrations has been utilized [21]. Recent studies at the M.D. Anderson Hospital yielded responses in 5 of 10 patients (50%). The degree of tumor necrosis varied from 70 to 100%.

Limb salvage is currently performed by two separate techniques. (1) Primary en bloc resection with insertion of a prefabricated endoprosthesi$. (2) Primary treatment with chemotherapy. This is followed by en bloc resection and insertion of a custom-made prosthesis.

Preoperative chemotherapy is administered to ablate the primary tumor and micrometastases. The approach, however, may be hazardous if chemotherapy is ineffective. The magnitude of the risk is unknown. Destruction of the primary tumor and microscopic disease may not be mutually exclusive: in each, the response may be influenced separately by pH, oxygenation, vascular supply, metabolic products and other factors. Recent reports would suggest that the hazard is minimal [36].

The efficacy of preoperative treatment is determined by clinical, radiographic and radionuclide parameters. Ultimately, however, the effect must be established by pathological examination. For this purpose, new criteria to determine response were developed [1, 36]. At the M.D. Anderson Hospital this involves a quantitative estimation of necrosis, degree of fibrosis with regeneration and tumor viability. The criteria are used in the selection of adjuvant chemotherapy after definitive surgery. Conceptually, this experience could lead to treatment based on tumor subtyping.

Ewing's Sarcoma

During the past decade, investigations have demonstrated that Ewing's sarcoma is sensitive to the following chemotherapeutic agents: vincristine, cyclophosphamide, actinomycin-D, adriamycin, BCNU and mithramycin. Combinations of these agents with different mechanisms of action and minimal overlapping toxicity have been employed to treat established disease and as adjuvant therapy. With current methods of treatment, the 3- to 5-year actuarial disease-free survival in localized disease has been escalated to 55–75% [5, 24, 35]. This must be compared with historical control patients in whom survival varied from 8 to 24% [2, 15].

Definitive treatment for Ewing's sarcoma is usually accomplished with radiation therapy. Megavoltage equipment and improved technique permit the safe administration of 4,500 rad in 4–4½ weeks. This includes generous coverage of all soft tissues likely to be infiltrated by tumor. Thereafter, 2,000 rad is administered over 2–2½ weeks to the radiographically determined area of involvement. Utilizing this approach with combination chemotherapy, local control and functional restoration can be anticipated in over 80% of patients [34].

Actinomycin-D and adriamycin augment the efficacy and toxicity of radiation. Combination treatment with these modalities, therefore, must be skillfully integrated. Delayed radiation complications include fractures of the irradiated bone, contractures of the irradiated limb and the emergence of second malignant neoplasms [28, 41].

The results in localized Ewing's sarcoma represent a major advance. However, they contrast sharply with those in patients presenting with metastatic disease in whom survival is probably less than 10%.

Non-Hodgkin's Lymphoma of Bone

Non-Hodgkin's lymphoma of the bone is an uncommon malignancy in childhood. The biologic behavior of the disease is similar to non-Hodgkin's lymphoma at other sites. It has a significant propensity to convert to acute leukemia. Published reports reveal a 35–50% 5-year survival [3, 32, 46]. The outlook for this desease, however, has changed with antileukemic combination chemotherapy and radiation administered to the primary tumor. Cure in over 80% of patients can be anticipated. [19].

Eosinophilic Granuloma

Solitary eosinophilic granuloma is usually treated by excisional curettage, biopsy or localized radiation. Recent investigations have demonstrated that direct injections of methyl prednisolone may also achieve cure [6]. The procedure produces immediate relief of pain, decrease in tumor size, sclerosis of the margins and progressive increase in trabeculation with filling in of the cavity. The mechanism of action is unknown. It represents an attractive therapeutic alternative to curettage and radiation which may damage an adjacent epiphyseal plate.

Refinements in Surgery

Advances achieved with chemotherapy, particularly in osteosarcoma, led to new dimensions in surgical treatment. There are currently 3 major surgical approaches. (1) Excisional biopsy. This includes curettage for benign or low grade tumors unlikely to recur. (2) Wide local resection with a cuff of normal tissue and bone adjacent to the tumor. It is employed in limb salvage and low grade malignent tumors, e.g., parosteal osteosarcoma. (3) Radical ablation. This involves amputation of disarticulation. The procedure is performed at a level sufficiently distant from the primary lesion to eliminate local spread throughout the medullary cavity or along tissue planes. It is used particularly to extirpate high grade tumors with a high propensity for metastasis.

The introduction of limb salvage entailed creation of specific eligibility criteria. These may be defined as follows. (1) Patients with lesions in the distal femur or proximal tibia must have maximum or near maximum growth. This is based upon the reconstruction technique. Resection of the tumor generally involves the knee epiphyses which precludes further growth. The predicted leg length discrepancy therefore should not exceed 8 cm. Alternatively, amputation using an exo-prosthesis would be preferable. (2) Patients with upper extremity lesions receive favorable consideration. In contrast to the lower extremity, lesions of the upper extremity will not produce a similar handicap. (3) Surgery should permit resection without sacrifice of a major vessel or nerve.

Limb salvage usually involves insertion of an internal prosthesis, coupled with total joint replacement. The prosthesis is manufactured from vitalium. Allograft tissues are generally not employed because of poor incorporation with postoperative chemotherapy. Custom-made prostheses usually permit satisfactory functional restoration and skeletal continuity. However, the future of these devices is uncertain particularly in young patients.

Immune Mechanisms

Attempts to increase or enhance immunologic responses of the host against the tumor have been investigated during the past decade. In osteosarcoma, studies suggest that interferon and transfer factor may have some promise [27, 40]. None of these methods, however, has demonstrated a clear-cut improvement over 'conventional' treatment with surgery and chemotherapy. Further investigation is required before they may be adopted as an important adjunct to treatment.

Controversial Issues

Advances achieved during the past decade have not been without controversy. The Mayo Clinic has criticized the use of historical controls in the osteosarcoma studies. It also reported a 40–50% disease-free survival during recent years without the potential benefit of adjuvant chemotherapy [12, 43]. This differs from previous reports published by this Institution where a 20% historical survival was similarly reported [10]. The controversy is bolstered by a report from Sweden claiming no survival differences between contemporary and historical control patients [4].

These differences are unresolved. However, they prompted some investigators to reevaluate their previous experiences and they again confirmed the validity of their historical controls [17, 31]. In addition, the observations reported from Sweden [4] were rebutted by *Gehan and Sutow* [18]. It was their contention that the Swedish study simply provided a description of patient characteristics which the authors failed to correlate with disease-free and overall survival. Further, *Gehan and Sutow* [18] asserted their belief that historical controls indeed constituted a valid basis for comparison since techniques were available to achieve reliability and adjust for differences in prognostic variables.

These controversial issues were useful and constructive. They generated studies which revealed that in analyzing survival, age, sex, primary site, histologic grade and tumor type must also be considered [9, 16, 18, 39]. The telangiectatic variety, for example, is characterized by an extremely unfavorable prognosis, whereas the low grade intermedullary type carries a more favorable outcome [29, 44]. Facial and jaw tumors also carry a better prognosis [26]. These developments are an inevitable result of new discoveries and must also be considered a sign of progress.

References

1   Ayala, A.G.; Mackay, B.; Jaffe, N.; Sutow, W.W.; Benjamin, R.; Murray, J.A.: Osteosarcoma. The pathological study of specimens from en bloc resection in patients receiving pro-operative chemotherapy; in van Eys, Sullivan, Status of the curability of childhood cancers, pp. 127–144 (Raven Press, New York, 1980).

2   Bhansali, S.K.; Desai, P.B.; Ewing's sarcoma observations on 107 cases. J. Bone Jt Surg. *45-A:*541–553 (1963).

3   Boston, H.C.; Dahlin, D.C.; Ivins, J.C.; et al.: Malignant lymphoma (so-called reticulum cell sarcoma) of bone. Cancer *34:*1131–1137 (1974).

4   Brostrom, L.A.; Apairsi, T.; Ingimarsson, S.N.; Sagergren, C.; Nilsonne, U.; Seronde, H.; Soderberg, G.: Can historical controls be used in current clinical trials in osteosarcoma? Metastasis and survival in a historical and a concurrent group. Int. J. Radiat. Oncol. Biol. Phys. *6:*1717–1721, 1980.

5   Chan, R.C.; Sutow, W.W.; Linberg, R.D.; Samuels, D.A.: Management and results of localized Ewing's sarcoma. Cancer *43:*1001–1006 (1979).

6   Cohen, M.; Zornosa, J.; Cangir, A.; Murray, J.A.; Wallace, S.: Direct injection of methlyprednisolone sodium succinate in the treatment of solidary eosinophilic granuloma of bone. Radiology *136:*289–293 (1980).

7   Cortes, E.P.; Holland, J.F.; Wang, J.J.; et al.: Doxoubicin in disseminated osteosarcoma. I. Am. med. Ass. *221:*1132–1138 (1972).

8   Cortes, E.P.; Holland, J.F.; Glidewell, O.: Amputation and adriamycin in primary osteosarcoma. A 5-year report. Cancer Treat. Rep. *62:*271–277 (1978).

9   Dahlin, D.C.: Osteosarcoma of bone and a consideration of prognostic variables. Cancer Treat. Rep. *62:*189–192 (1978).

10 Dahlin, D.C.; Coventry, M.B.: Osteogenic sarcoma. A study of 600 cases. J. Bone Jt Surg. *49:*101–110 (1967).

11 de Santos, L.A.; Bernadino, M.E.; Murray, J.A.: Sarcoma: experience with 25 cases. Am. J. Roentg. Rad. Ther. nucl. Med. *132:*535–560 (1979).

12 Edmonson, J.H.; Green, S.J.; Ivins, J.C.; Gilchrist, G.S.; Gregan, E.T.; Pritchard, D.J.; Smithson, W.A.; Dahlin, D.C.; Taylor, W.F.: Methotrexate as adjuvant treatment for primary osteosarcoma. New Engl. J.Med. *303:*642–645 (1980).

13 Eilber, F.R.; Morton, D.L.; Grant, T.T.: En bloc resection and allograft replacement for osteosarcoma of the extremity; in Jaffe, Bone tumors in children (PSG Publishing Co., Littleton, 1979).

14 Ettinger, L.J.; Douglass, H./., Jr.; Higby, I.J.; Mindell, E.R.; Nime, F.; Ghoorah, J.; Freeman, A.: Adjuvant adriamycin and cis-diammine-dichloroplatinum (cis-platinum) in primary osteosarcoma. Cancer *47:*248–254 (1981).

15 Falk, S.; Alpert: Five year survival of patients with Ewing's sarcoma. Surgery Gynec. Obstet. *124:*319–324 (1967).

16 Frei, E.; Jaffe, N.; Gero, M.; Skipper, H.; Watts; H.: Adjuvant chemotherapy of osteogenic sarcoma. Progress and perspectives. J. natn. Cancer Inst. *60:* 3–10 (1978).

17 Gehan, E.A.; Sutow, W.W.; Uribe-Botero, T.; Romsdahl, M.; Smith, T.L.: Osteosarcoma. The M.D. Anderson experience 1950–1974; in Terry, Windhorst, Immunotherapy of cancer. Present status of trials in man, pp. 271–282. (Raven Press, New York, 1978).

18 Gehan, E.A.; Sutow, W.W.: Evaluation of results of new treatments for osteosarcoma. Int. J. Radiat. Oncol. Biol. Phys. *6:*1757–1758 (1980).

19 Jaffe, N.; Buell, D.; Cassady, J.R.; et al.: The role of staging in non-Hodgkin's lymphoma of childhood. Cancer Treat. Rep. *61:*1001–1007 (1977).

20 Jaffe, N.; Watts, H.: Multidrug chemotherapy in primary treatment of osteosarcoma. J. Bone Jt Surg. *58-A/5:*634–635 (1976).

21   Jaffe, N.; Chuang, V.; Wallace, S.; Ayala, A.; Murray, J.; Romsdahl, M.; Benjamin, R.S.: Osteosarcoma: Control of the Primary Tumor with Intra-Arterial Cis-Di-aminedichloro Platinum II (IACDP) (Abstract 791). Proc. AACR/ASCO *21:* 797 (1980).

22   Jaffe, N.; Farber, S.; Traggis, D.; Geiser, C.; Kim, B.S.; Das, L.; Frauenberger, A.; Djerassi, I.; Cassady, J.R.: Favorable response of metastatic osteogic sarcoma to pulse high-dose methotrexate with citrovorum rescue and radiation therapy. Cancer *31:* 1367–1373 (1973).

23   Jaffe, N.; Link, M.; Traggis, D.; Frei, E.; Watts, H.; Beardsley, P.; Cohen, D.; Abelson, H.: The role of high dose methotrexate in osteogenic sarcoma. J. natn. Cancer Inst. (in press, 1979).

24   Jaffe, N.; Traggis, D.; Sallan, S.; Cassady, J.R.: Improved outlook for Ewing's sarcoma with combination chemotherapy (vincristine, adriamycin and cyclophosphamide) and radiation therapy. Cancer *38:* 1925–1930 (1976).

25   Jaffe, n.; Watts, H.; Fellows, K.E.; Vawter, C.: Local en bloc resection for limb preservation. Cancer Treat. Rep. *62:* 217–223 (1978).

26   Kragh, LV.; Dahlin, D.C.; Erich, J.B.: Osteogenic sarcoma of the jaws and facial bones. Am. J. Surg. *96:* 496–505 (1958).

27   Levin, A.S.; Beyer, V.S.; Fudenberg, H.H.; Wybran, J.; Hackett, A.J.; Johnston, J.O.; Spitler, L.L.: Osteogenic sarcoma. Immunotherapy with tumor specific transfer factor. J. clin. Invest. *55:* 487–499 (1975).

28   Lewis, R.J.; Marcove, R.C.; Rosen, G.: Ewing's sarcoma. Functional effects of radiation therapy. J. Bone Jt Surg. *59:* 325–331 (1977).

29   Matsuno, T.; Unni, K.K.; McLeod, R.A.; et al.: Telangiectatic osteogenic sarcoma. Cancer *38:* 2538–2547 (1976).

30   McNeil, B.J.; Cassady, J.R.; Geiser, C.F.; Jaffe, N.; Traggis, D.; Treves, S.: Fluorine-18 bone scintigraphy in children with osteosarcoma or Ewings's sarcoma. Radiology *109:* 627–631 (1973).

31   Mike, V.; Marcove, R.C.: Osteogenic sarcoma under the age of 21. Experiences at Memorial Sloan-Kettering Cancer Center; in Terry, Windhorst, Immunotherapy of cancer. Present status of trials in man, pp. 283–292 (Raven Press, New York, 1978).

32   Newall, J.; Friedman, M.; Navaez, F.: Extralymph-node reticulum cell sarcoma. Radiology *91:* 708–712 (1968).

33   Ochs, J.J.; Freeman, A.I.; Douglass, H.O., Jr.; Higby, D.J.; Mindell, E.R.; Sinks, T.: Cis-dichloro-diammine platinum (II) in advanced osteogenic sarcoma. Cancer Treat. Rep. *62:* 239–245 (1978).

34   Perez, C.A.; Razak, M.; Tefft, M.; Nesbit, O.; Burgert, J.; Kissone, T.; Vietti, T.; Gehan, E.A.: Analysis of local control in Ewing's sarcoma. Cancer *40:* 2864–2873 (1977).

35   Rosen, G.; Caparros, B.; Mosende, C.; et al.: Curability of Ewing's sarcoma and considerations for future therapeutic trials. Cancer *41:* 888–899 (1978).

36   Rosen, G.; Marcove, R.C.; Caparros, B.; Nirenberg, A.; Kosloff, C.; Huvos, A.G.: Primary osteogenic sarcoma. The rationale for preoperative chemotherapy and delayed surgery. Cancer *43:* 2163–2177 (1979).

37   Rosen, G.; Murphy, M.L.; Huvos, A.G.; Gutierrez, M.; Marcove, C.: Chemotherapy, en bloc resection, and prosthetic bone replacement in the treatment of osteogenic sarcoma. Cancer *37:* 1–11 (1976).

38 Rosen, G.; Nirenberg, A.; Juergens, H.; Kosloff, B.; Mehta, B.M.; Marcove, R.C.; Huvos, A.G.: Osteogenic sarcoma. Three year disease free survival in excess of 80% with combination chemotherapy including effective high dose methotrexate with citrovorum factor rescue. J. natn. Cancer Inst. (in press, 1979).

39 Simon, R.: Clinical prognostic factors in osteosarcoma. Cancer Treat. Rep. *62:* 193–197 (1978).

40 Strander, H.: Antitumor effects of interferon and its possible use as an antineoplastic agent in man. Tex. Rep. Biol. Med. *35:* 629–635 (1977).

41 Strong, L.G.; Herson, G.H.; Osborne, B.M.; Sutow, W.W.: Risk of radiation related malignant tumor in survivors of Ewing's sarcoma. J. natn. Cancer Inst. *62:* 1401–1405 (1979).

42 Sutow, W.W.; Gehan, E.A.; Vietti, T.J.; Frias, A.E.; Dyment, P.G.: Multidrug chemotherapy in primary treatment of osteosarcoma. J. Bone Jt Surg. *58-A:* 629–633 (1976).

43 Taylor, W.F.; Ivins, J.G.; Dahlin, D.C.; Pritchard, O.J.: Osteogenic sarcoma experience at the Mayo Clinic 1963–1974 in immunotherapy of cancer; in Terry, Windhorst, Present status of trials in man, pp. 257–269 (Raven press, New York, 1978).

44 Unni, K.K.; Dahlin, D.C.; Beabout, J.W.; et al.: Parosteal osteogenic sarcoma. Cancer *37:* 2466–2475 (1976).

45 Wallace, S.; Granmayeh, M.; L.A. de Santos; Murray, J.A.; Romsdahl, M.M.; Bracken, R.B.; Jansson, K.: Arterial occlusion of pelvic bone tumors. Cancer *43:* 322–328 (1979).

46 Wang, C.C.; Fletcher, D.J.: Primary reticulum cell sarcoma of bone. Cancer *22:* 994–998 (1968).

N. Jaffe, MD, Department of Pediatrics,
M.D. Anderson Hospital and Tumor Institute, Houston, TX 77030 (USA)

Front. Radiat. Ther. Onc., vol. 16, pp. 114–121 (Karger, Basel 1982)

Soft Tissue Sarcomas in Childhood

Daniel M. Hays

USC School of Medicine, Children's Hospital of Los Angeles, Los Angeles, Calif., USA

General Considerations

Although sarcoma of soft tissue is uncommon, viz. 4,500 newly diagnosed patients per year in the US population, there has been an increase in general medical interest in the problem of managing patients with the condition because of new strategies of management and improvement in clinical results.

The term 'soft tissue sarcoma' has been confined to extremity (or trunk and extremity) lesions by some; however, tumors with similar histology occur in the viscera, constituting in many cases the most significant group of tumors of this type. We will include all sites and all tumor types which might be included in this category, except for nephroblastoma and neuroblastoma.

The unique aspects of the surgical management of sarcomas in childhood are the results of two factors: (a) some sarcomas (fibrosarcomas) in infants or young children have many of the characteristics of benign tumors, despite a malignant histologic appearance, and during these early years may be managed by more conservative surgical approaches; (b) some sarcomas (rhabdomyosarcoma) have shown such marked sensitivity to chemotherapeutic agents (or chemotherapy/radiotherapy) that surgical and radiotherapy approaches to these tumors have been radically modified. This sensitivity is apparently influenced by histologic type and subtype as well as site. It should be stressed that major treatment decisions in childhood should be made after a detailed histologic examination is completed and this is rarely possibly on the basis of rapid section study.

This group of tumors was long regarded as relatively radioresistant but employing modern techniques they can be locally controlled with appropriate dosage. One advantage of radiation therapy is the ease with which the treatment volume can be designated to include tissues suspected of involvement without concern for position of nerve, vessels, or tendons; i.e., the treatment volume can be extended in certain critical dimensions much easier than can the surgical treatment volume. The major effects of radiotherapy on bone growth in the extremities during childhood may influence decisions regarding the therapy plan.

In certain specific types and sites chemotherapy has become the paramount therapy modality, and changes in surgery and radiotherapy have been adaptive. This sensitivity, however, is variable, and in other situations, surgery and radiotherapy play the major role influencing survival. A combined therapy approach is essential.

The following sections concentrate on those areas in which somewhat unique therapeutic procedures are employed in the management of soft tissue sarcomas in childhood.

Rhabdomyosarcoma

General Remarks
Symptoms alerting the physician to the presence of this sarcoma are extremely diverse because it may occur in any body site. The head and neck region and lower genitourinary tract are usually affected in infants and small children; while in adolescents, trunk, extremity, and paratesticular sites are common.

Chemotherapy, initially an adjuvant to surgery and radiation, has become the primary form of therapy in the more responsive types of rhabdomyosarcomas. In these patients, surgery may take the form of a radical local excision, in an area free of significant structures; or a simple gross excision, when removal of an important organ or structure would be required by a radical approach. Surgery has also been used to reduce tumor bulk prior to intensive chemotherapy and to remove residual tumor after a successful chemotherapy (or chemotherapy/radiotherapy) regimen.

All patients with rhabdomyosarcoma should be treated with combination chemotherapy. The best regimen, however, free of significant toxicity, has yet to be developed. The drugs most active against rhabdomyosarcoma are vincristine, dactinomycin, cyclophosphamide, and adriamycin, and they are best administered in 2–4 drug combinations.

In the subsequent paragraphs, the results of the (U.S.) Intergroup Rhabdomyosarcoma Study, IRS, are the source of data, and also of the staging system employed.

At the present time, the basic approach to chemotherapy is the use of less intensive chemotherapy regimens for patients with no residual disease (group I) or microscopic residual disease (group II) following surgery, with more intensive schedules reserved for patients with gross residual (group III) or metastatic (group IV) disease at diagnosis, emphasizing the critical role of accurate staging. The relapse-free survival rates at 3 years by group are: group I, 83%; II, 66%; III, 57%; IV, 29%; all patients having received VAC (vincristine, dactinomycin, cyclophosphamide) combinations with or without adriamycin and radiation therapy postoperatively. 25% of the patients who receive standard VAC therapy preoperatively achieve a complete response by 6 weeks. After radiation therapy is administered to these patients at 6 weeks, the complete response rate increases to 50% and the partial response rate increases to 30% for an overall favorable response rate of 80%.

Rhabdomyosarcomas of the trunk and extremities have not responded to chemotherapy regimens as dramatically as have those in the genitourinary track or even the head and neck sites [6]. Radical surgical procedures are probably indicated for all tumors in these areas.

Primary Pelvic Rhabdomyosarcomas

These sarcomas, arising in the bladder, prostate, and female genital tract have always represented major problems in management, and are a source of intense emotional stress for parents and involved physicians. Remarkable improvement relative to survival resulted from the adoption of a combined therapy approach including pelvic exenteration and an intensive radiotherapy/chemotherapy regimen [1]. As the long-range psychic and social impact of pelvic exenteration in this age group was fully appreciated, these results seemed less impressive. New approaches are almost entirely attempts to avoid exenteration.

For two decades chemotherapy has been employed before definitive surgery in children believed to have localized but 'unresectable' rhabdomyosarcomas in the pelvis and elsewhere. The aim of this approach was to reduce the volume of the tumor with chemotherapy, followed when feasible by exterpative surgery (and radiotherapy). Some of these patients have had extended tumor-free survival. Others with pelvic primaries have required diversion of the urinary tract because of bladder malfunction secondary to irradiation, chemotherapy, and surgery; despite local tumor control.

More recently a similar approach has been adopted in patients that have pelvic rhabdomyosarcomas which are apparently 'resectable' (by exenteration) or those in which resectability is not determined. Following endoscopic biopsy these children are initially placed on an intensive chemotherapy regimen (usually 'pulse' VAC) frequently combined with radiotherapy, with the hope of limiting the scope of surgery. Effective long-range multiple-agent chemotherapy is the essential component of this approach. Results of clinical trials in this area, i.e., 'primary' chemotherapy for pelvic rhabdomyosarcoma [5, 10, 12] may be summarized as follows: Female infants with tumors primary of the vulva, vagina, or cervix usually respond to chemotherapy and the rate of survival has been >80% as determined by combining reported and other available series. Intensive chemotherapy for a period of 3–6 months is ordinarily followed by elective partial vaginectomy and simple hysterectomy to remove possible residual tumor. Chemotherapy is then resumed. ovarian function was at least partially retained in most patients. Pelvic exenteration was required for failure of response (<20%) or relapse.

In some patients with bladder rhabdomyosarcomas located outside of the trigone area, tumor removal by partial cystectomy has been possible; and in some series, more than half of these patients are surviving without recurrence. Bladder lesions situated in the trigone region, and the primary prostatic rhabdomyosarcomas are treated by repeated endoscopic partial excisions. Approximately 60% of these have responded to a primary chemotherapy regimen, usually combined with radiotherapy. Postresponse prostatectomy (not exenteration) has also been employed.

There is a significant group of patients who do not respond to either primary chemotherapy or a chemotherapy/radiotherapy regimen (15–25% in most series) and these should be treated by pelvic exenteration. Patients who have *not* responded to a primary chemotherapy regimen over a 6-month period and had subsequent pelvic exenteration are alive and without relapse.

Few of the reported series in which a primary chemotherapy/radiotherapy regimen has been employed have been in existence long enough to provide a valid concept of long-range survival. It would appear, however, that the primary chemotherapy regimens have been initially successful in approximately 70% of these patients. Following failure of the regimen, exenteration and extended survival also appears to be probable. It should be noted that the primary chemotherapy regimens have been less successfully applied to the nonpelvic sites.

Rhabdomyosarcomas of Other Sites

Orbital rhabdomyosarcomas are usually treated by biopsy and radiotherapy, with or without chemotherapy, with a survival rate of approximately 90%. Other primary head and neck rhabdomyosarcomas, when superficial, may be exised; and this should be carried out when feasible, as patients in which a gross resection of the tumor is accomplished have the highest survival rates. However, the majority of these patients must be treated by biopsy, radiotherapy, and intensive chemotherapy. Even in these, survival rates are approximately 50%. Patients with parameningeal lesions of the head and neck area, who are at risk of developing meningeal disease, should be given intrathecal chemotherapy in addition to cranial irradiation. The results obtained thus far in IRS-II support this recommendation.

Particularly low survival rates have been seen in patients with primary lesions of the retroperitoneal space, perineum, and perianal regions [7]. In these areas, radical surgical procedures should be encouraged, as well as intensive local radiotherapy and chemotherapy regimens, as survival rates remain low [4>.

The importance of the alveolar subtype in adversely influencing survival in all sites is noted. Whether this should influence the type of surgical procedure performed is questionable, as in general, relapse in patients with this particularly *lethal* subtype have been distant, rather than local. All forms of therapy should be energetically employed in this subgroup of children with rhabdomyosarcomas.

Fibrosarcoma

Congenital fibrosarcomas, and those appearing during the first several years of life have been recognized to have benign characteristics despite similar histologic features to those seen in adults [2, 11]. In congenital forms metastasis is extremely uncommon, despite high rates of local recurrence.

Most smaller fibrosarcomas are excised without preliminary biopsy and the tumor type and histologic features are unknown at the time of surgery. Despite 'inadequate' cancer surgery, most of these patients, i.e., infants and small children with fibrosarcoma, do not develop local recurrence. This is true even in tumors with an antaplastic or 'invasive' histologic appearance. Tumor recurrence, when it occurs, is treated more agressively surgically and may eventually lead to amputation or other radical procedures.

Early life is also the period of the greatest diagnostic confusion in respect to the histology of these tumors, which must be differentiated by pathologists [3], from the larger group of tumors which may be collectively termed 'fascial fibromatosis'. This fact, also, dictates conservatism in surgery as misdiagnosis is common.

Beyond the age of 10, this surgical conservatism must be modified, and patients over 15 should be treated as adults. The same limb-saving procedures employed in adults can be considered, but almost full skeletal growth must be obtained before these are applicable to pediatric patients, particularly in the care of lesions of the lower extremities.

Synovial Sarcomas (Malignant Synovioma)

The classical history of this disease is one of repeated local recurrence, but dissemination occurs earlier and more frequently than in fibrosarcoma. These tumors occur late in childhood or in young adults and are most frequently in the lower extremities. A special problem in the younger children arises when the lesion is adjacent to the osseous growth centers adjacent to the knee. If total removal by wide local excision is not possible in such cases, amputation may be preferable to a limited resection and high dose radiation therapy. Limb shortening after radiation therapy in prepubertal children presents major orthopedic problems.

Small Cell Soft Tissue Sarcoma (Extra-Osseous 'Ewing's Sarcoma')

These tumors are usually found in older children and largely confined to the musculature of the trunk and extremity. In the past, they have been treated by radical surgical procedures, usually without survival. Many were consciously or inadvertently included on the chemotherapy regimens of rhabdomyosarcoma studies, and have responded to treatment by VAC or similar regimens.

Hemangiopericytoma

This highly malignant soft tissue tumor was formerly only occassionally managed effectively by radical excision. It has been recently recognized that the size of the primary tumor may frequently be reduced and metastasis may be controlled by chemotherapy [8]. These tumors are usually initially nonresectable, but may be removed at a secondary procedure following response to chemotherapy.

Neurofibrosarcoma

Neurofibromata are common in childhood, but malignancy appears in less than 10% of this group of patients. Neurofibrosarcomas also appear in children without a history of neurofibromatosis. When multiple, neurofibromata are managed by conservative local excisions. It has been felt that malignant forms were quite unresponsive to radiotherapy and chemotherapy, but recent results suggest that control can be achieved with an aggressive multimodality approach including initial radical surgery [9].

References

1   Clatworthy, H.W., Jr.; Braren, V.; Smith, J.P.: Surgery of bladder and prostatic neoplasms in children. Cancer *32:* 1157 (1973).
2   Exelby, R.P.; et al.: Soft-tissue fibrosarcoma in children. J. pediat. Surg. *8:* 415 (1973).
3   Hays, D.M.; Mirabal, V.Q.; Karlan, M.S.; Patel, H.R.; Landing, B.H.: Fibrosarcomas in infants and children. J. pediat. Surg. *5:* 176–183 (1970).
4   Hays, D.M.: The management of rhabdomyosarcoma in children and young adults. Wld J. Surg. *4:* 15–28 (1980).
5   Kumar, A.P.M.; et al.: Combined therapy to prevent complete pelvic exenteration for rhabdomyosarcoma of the vagina or uterus. Cancer *37:* 118 (1976).

6   Maurer, H.M.: Rhabdomyosarcoma in childhood and adolescence. Curr. Prob. Cancer *2:* 3–36 (1978).

7   Maurer, H.M.; Donaldson, M.; Gehan, E.A.; Hammond, D.; Hays, D.M.; Lawrence W., Jr.; Lindberg, R.; Newton, W.; Ragab, A.; Raney, R.B., Jr.; Ruymann, F.; Soule, E.H.; Sutow, W.W.; Tefft, M. (for the IRS Committee): The intergroup rhabdomyosarcoma study. Update – November 1978. J. natn. Cancer Inst. (in press).

8   Ortega, J.A.; et al.: Chemotherapy of malignant hemangiopericytoma of childhood. Cancer *27:* 730 (1971).

9   Raney, R.B., Jr.; Littman, P.S.; Jarrett, P.; Waldman, M.T.G.; Chatter, J.: Results of multi-modal therapy for children with neurogenic sarcoma. Med. Pediat. Oncol. (in press).

10 Rivard, G.; et al.: Intensive chemotherapy as primary treatment for rhabdomyosarcoma of the pelvis. Cancer *36:* 1593 (1975).

11 Soule, E.H.; Prichard, D.J.: Fibrosarcoma in infants and children. A review of 110 cases. Cancer *40:* 1711 (1977).

12 Voute, A.P.; Vos, A.: Combination chemotherapy as primary treatment in children with rhabdomyosarcoma to avoid mutilating surgery or radiotherapy (Abstract). Proc. 13th Ann. Meet. Am. Soc. clin. Oncol. *18:* 327 (1977).

D.M. Hays, MD, Professor of Surgery, USC School of Medicine,
Children's Hospital of Los Angeles, Los Angeles, CA 90033 (USA)

Front. Radiat. Ther. Onc., vol. 16, pp. 122–133 (Karger, Basel 1982)

Hodgkin's Disease

Treatment with Low Dose Radiation and Chemotherapy[1]

Sarah S. Donaldson

Department of Radiology, Division of Radiation Therapy, Stanford University
School of Medicine, Stanford, Calif., USA

During the past 2 decades, major medical advances have resulted
in dramatic improvements in cure rates for the majority of children
with cancer, including those with Hodgkin's disease. Although it was
once thought that children with Hodgkin's disease displayed characteristics that differed significantly from adults similarly afflicted, and that
children faired less well than adults [27], these notions have not been
confirmed in more recent analyses [10, 18]. When looking at the influence of age upon prognosis, *Kaplan* [18] has shown that patients 15
years of age or less have a prognosis comparable to those in the 17–49
age range, and have a significantly improved liklihood of cure when
compared to a population 50 years of age or older. In addition, the
response to MOPP chemotherapy [7] correlates directly with the age of
the patient. *Coltman* [4] and SWOG investigators demonstrated significantly improved survival among children less than 20 years of age
treated with MOPP alone, as compared to patients in the age range 20–
40, 40–60, or greater than 60 years of age.

Thus, there is now increasing evidence to support the fact that
children with Hodgkin's disease can be compared favorably to adults
with the disease. However, whereas the biology, natural history, and
response to treatment of Hodgkin's disease in children is similar to the
disease in the adult population, children do differ from adults in that
complications from therapy can be more serious and severe in this

[1] Supported in part by Public Health Service Research grant CA 05838 from the
National Cancer Institute, National Institutes of Health, Bethesda, USA.

growing population. Thus, children with Hodgkin's disease present therapeutic dilemmas when one is faced with options regarding treatment programs.

Results of Therapy

Large series of carefully staged and treated children with Hodgkin's disease now reveal 5-year survival rates of 92–93% and 5-year relapse-free survival rates ranging from 57 to 82% when pathologic staging is uniformly used [10, 17]. The Boston series of 52 children with pathologic stage I–III disease reveals 90% of patients continously free of disease and 98% alive without evidence of disease at a median follow-up interval of 3 years [1]. Those children with pathologic stage I and IIA disease were treated with high dose extended field irradiation, those with stage IIIA disease with total nodal irradiation, and those with systemic symptoms with total nodal irradiation plus MOPP.

Long-term data from Stanford reveals actuarial 5-, 10- and 15-year survival rates of 90, 80 and 70% and corresponding freedom from relapse rates of 75, 66 and 66%, respectively [11]. Although most relapses occur within the first 3 years following diagnosis, late relapses as long as 8 years following initial treatment have occurred among children not surgically staged or in whom no subdiaphragmatic irradiation was given [11]. *Jenkin and Berry* [17] have reported 10-year survival and relapse-free survival rates of 89 and 54% in children with Hodgkin's disease. Their patients who relapsed were generally treated with MOPP chemotherapy and supplemental irradiation. These authors made the observation that salvage therapy was effective in their hands in maintaining a median duration of second remission of only 3 years, with more than half of the children who experienced an initial relapse, suffering multiple relapses. Such observations support the concept of utilizing combined modality therapy as initial treatment for those with advanced disease, rather than relying on radiation alone with salvage chemotherapy if necessary.

The radiotherapy results support the use of radiation as single modality therapy for patients with pathologic stage IA, IIA, IB, IIB, and subsets of patients with IIIA disease, if one is willing to utilize high doses ($\pm$ 4,400 rad) and extended fields [14]. Whereas such a program can indeed be curative in children with Hodgkin's disease, if one can avoid the known sequelae of high dose irradiation [25] without compromising the results of treatment in growing children, it is advantageous to do so. MOPP chemotherapy alone has been used at the Uganda Cancer Institute in Kampala for children with Hodgkin's disease where radiation therapy facilities are nonexistent [21]. Whereas 88% of children can be expected to achieve a complete remission, with 74% remaining in first remission at 5 years from MOPP therapy, the 5-year survival rate for the entire group is only 67%. Approximately 75% of children with clinical stage I and II disease will survive at 5 years, but only 60% of those with stage III and IV disease [21]. Similar results in America have been reported by *Coltman* [4].

The group at Princess Margaret Hospital in Toronto introduced a policy of using involved field radiation for children with clinical stage I disease, and extended field radiation and 6 cycles of MOPP chemotherapy for those with stage II–IV disease [16, 17]. Since all children received systemic chemotherapy, pathologic staging was not employed. They have used extended field treatment including mantle and para-aortic fields in doses in the range of 2,000–3,500 rad, reporting a 5-year survival rate of 89% and relapse-free survival rate of 85% among 41 children [17]. They have noted that 4 of 9 children with clinical stage IVB disease have relapsed using this regimen making the relapse-free survival less than 50% for this unfavorable group of children.

Stanford Protocol of Low Dose Radiation + Chemotherapy

The present challenge in the treatment of children with Hodgkin's disease is to delineate a therapeutic program which will insure continuation of the excellent survival and disease-free survival figures which are now being achieved while minimizing the risks of complications from treatment. An area of great concern in young children is the impairment of bone growth and development which is known to accompany high dose large volume radiation [22, 23, 26]. 12 years ago *Kaplan* devised a pilot program at Stanford designed to ascertain if multiple cycles of MOPP chemotherapy could be used to replace a portion of the needed radiation dose in pathologic staged children with Hodgkin's disease. Since that time 48 children have been treated at Stanford with low dose radiotherapy and MOPP. The protocol utilized is shown in table I. All children receive 6 cycles of MOPP chemother-

Table I. Stanford pediatric Hodgkin's disease protocol

Pathologic stage[1]	Treatment: radiation and chemotherapy
IA, IIA	involved field and MOPP ×6
I_EA, II_EA	subtotal lymphoid and MOPP ×6
IB, IIB	total lymphoid and MOPP ×6
I_EB, II_EB	total lymphoid and MOPP ×6
IIIA, III_EA, III_SA	total lymphoid and MOPP ×6
IIIB, III_EB, III_SB	alternating MOPP and radiotherapy[2]
Multiple E, IV	alternating MOPP and radiotherapy[2]
IV_M	MOPP ×6, radiotherapy, and maintenance MOPP
Radiation dose	
Bone age	
Less than 6 years	1,500 rad
6–10 years	2,000 rad
11–14 years	2,500 rad
MOPP dose	
Nitrogen mustard, 6 mg/m² i.v. days 1, 8	
Vincristine, 1.4 mg/m² i.v. days 1, 8 (limit 2 mg)	
Procarbazine, 100 mg/m² p.o. days 2–14	
Prednisone, 40 mg/m² p.o. days 1–14 with rapid tapering, cycles 1 and 4; omit in children who receive mantle irradiation	

[1] Ann Arbor staging [2].

[2] MOPP × 2 cycles followed by radiotherapy to one region, followed by MOPP × 2 cycles, followed by radiotherapy to a second region, with a total at 6 cycles of MOPP, as described by *Hoppe* et al. [15].

apy and radiation to at least known sites of disease. As the administered radiation volumes are determined by pathologic staging, all children undergo staging laparotomy with splenectomy. The given dose of radiation is decreased as low as 1,500 rad for youngsters less than 6 years of age; the volume of radiation reduced to involved fields in those children known to have localized disease confirmed by a negative staging laparotomy with splenectomy.

The actuarial analysis of survival and freedom from relapse are 96% and 93%, respectively, as shown in figure 1. There have been only 3 relapses. Two of these occurred in children presenting with extensive stage IV disease including bone marrow involvement who failed to respond to MOPP chemotherapy, were never disease-free, and died within 6 months of diagnosis. In contrast those with stage IV liver or

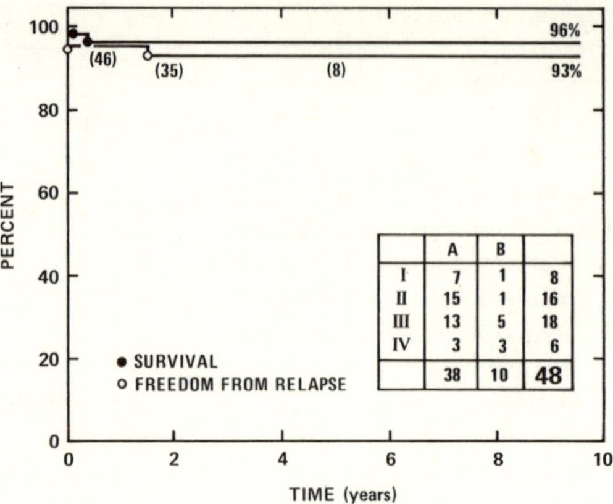

	A	B	
I	7	1	8
II	15	1	16
III	13	5	18
IV	3	3	6
	38	10	48

Fig. 1. Actuarial analysis by the method of Kaplan and Meier of survival and freedom from relapse among 48 children treated with low-dose irradiation and MOPP. The stages of the children are shown in the insert.

lung disease have faired much better to this approach than those presenting with bone marrow involvement. The third relapse occurred in a girl with stage $III_{EE}B$ disease involving the lung and pericardium. She recurred at 18 months in an irradiated neck node, received further radiation and has no evidence of disease at present. As the maximum follow-up of this group is 10 years, with median follow-up of only 3 years, longer evaluation is necessary to ascertain the ultimate disease status and complications of treatment.

Figure 2 shows the anatomic distribution of 215 sites of involvement of various lymphatic and extra lymphatic sites at the time of presentation among these 48 surgically staged children with Hodgkin's disease. Although not common, involvement of Waldeyer's ring does occur thus necessitating careful inspection of this area. Epitrochlear, bracheal and popliteal adenopathy are rare and did not occur among this series of children. Supradiaphragmatic disease is common with nearly 80% of children presenting with disease in one or both necks. Extranodal extension to the pericardium, pleura and pulmonary parenchyma is most often observed in the presence of massive mediastinal and/or hilar disease.

Figure 3 shows the status of control of 159 involved lymph node regions in these 48 children. Sites were scored as involved on the basis of palpable disease considered positive by physical examination and

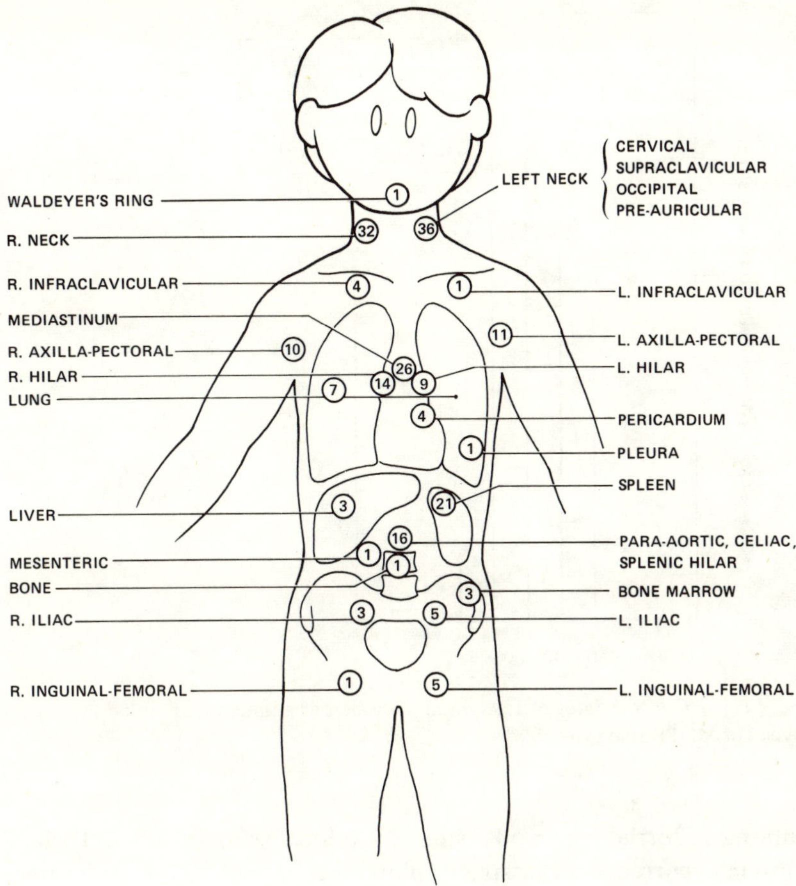

Fig. 2. Anatomic distribution of 215 lymphatic and extralymphatic sites of documented involvement among 48 surgically staged children with Hodgkin's disease.

on radiographic extent of disease as determined by chest X-ray, whole lung tomograms, and lymphangiogram; each lymph node region was scored individually as in the Ann Arbor staging system [19]. Patients were randomized to receive 1,500, 2,000 or 2,500 rad on the basis of their bone age as shown in table I. However, massive lymphadenopathy not overlying the axial skeleton has been locally boosted to 3,000–3,500 rad in select patients with persistent adenopathy after radiation and/or MOPP chemotherapy. There has been only 1 relapse

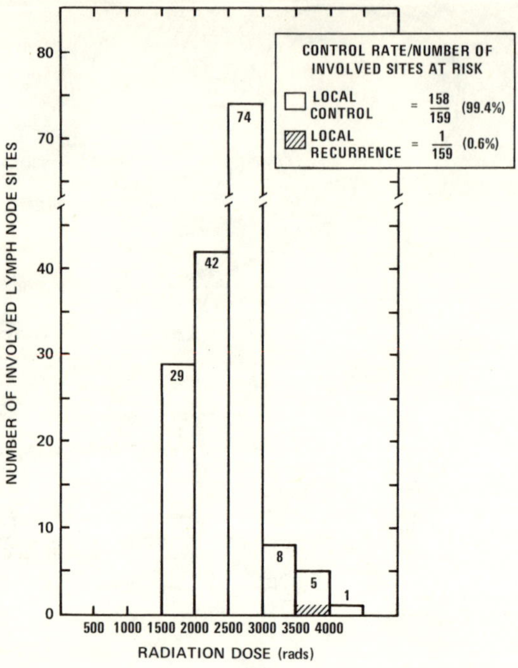

Fig. 3. Control status of 159 lymph node sites as a function of radiation dose and 6 cycles of MOPP among 48 children.

among 159 irradiated nodal sites, for a local relapse rate of 0.6%. This failure occurred in a massively enlarged cluster of lymph nodes treated to 3,500 rad plus 6 cycles of MOPP.

Complications of Treatment

The recognized limitations of aggressive combined modality therapy for Hodgkin's disease have been described well [8, 9, 11, 18, 25, 26]. In a pediatric population undergoing active growth and development, the known sequelae to growing bone and soft tissue, and to organ, endocrine and gonadal function can be expected to be more severe than in an adult population in which growth and development has largely been completed by the time of treatment. The impact of therapy upon children is even greater when one considers that 90% of such children will be cured with expected longevity in excess of 50–60 years from the time of treatment.

The late effects of irradiation are directly related to dose and volume and inversely related to age of the child at the time of treatment. The marked bone growth effects of high dose total lymphoid irradiation results in disproportionate alteration in sitting height as compared to standing height. This abnormality is most marked in children less than 6 years of age or those in adolescence at the time of treatment, during which time bone growth is particularly active. Other resulting abnormalities may include a small thorax, short clavicles, narrow shoulders, and atrophy of the soft tissues of the neck as well as the effect on the axial skeleton [22, 23, 26].

Injury to organ function such as the heart and lung is related to the dose of radiation administered and to the techniques utilized. Such injury has been greatly minimized by refinements in the techniques of irradiation [9, 18]. The effects of endocrine abnormality can largely be avoided by attention to thyroid function and early use of replacement therapy. Gonadal shielding including oophoropexy as well as testicular shielding can reduce radiation exposure to sensitive gonadal structures to within limits compatible with fertility.

The complications relating to chemotherapy are just now being recognized [13], and require careful attention and long-term follow-up. Of great concern is the recognized influence of multiple agent chemotherapy on gonadal function. Ugandan adolescent boys with Hodgkin's disease treated with full courses of MOPP have been reported to develop moderate to severe gynecomastia, germinal aplasia, increased FSH and LH levels and decreased testosterone levels [24]. However, prepubertal Ugandan boys did not develop gynecomastia or changes in gonadotropin levels. Experience with adult males reveal that the probability of recovery of spermatogenic function and fertility is low following full courses of MOPP. An insufficient number of prepubertal boys have been treated and followed for a sufficient interval to determine if delayed effects to this population will be different from that of adolescent or adult males.

Of greatest concern in selection of treatment regimens for children with a high probability of long-term survival is the risk of a second malignant tumor following successful treatment of the first. The second neoplasms which have been reported have largely been hematopoetic malignancies and have been refractory to therapy. The incidence of developing AML is approximately 4% and non-Hodgkin's lymphoma 8% following high dose total lymphoid irradiation plus MOPP chemotherapy, and both incidences appear to be rising at 7 years [3, 20]. In the Stanford pediatric series 2.3% of children developed a second malignant tumor [11]. These have arisen exclusively in children receiving combined modality therapy including high dose large volume radiation and full courses of chemotherapy. These tumors include acute monocytic leukemia, non-Hodgkin's lymphoma, and two sarcomas. The subset at greatest risk appears to be those children treated initially with radiotherapy who have relapsed and required chemotherapy for salvage, as the incidence of second tumor is 8% among this unfortunate group of children [11].

The therapeutic plan of the Stanford pediatric protocol with low dose radiation and chemotherapy has greatly reduced the previously recognized complications attributed to high dose extended field irradiation. The acute morbidity of the protocol has been related to nausea and vomiting, peripheral neuropathy, hair loss, and bone marrow suppression from chemotherapy. These have all been reversible and not considered severe. Early thyroid dysfunction following irradiation doses of less than 2,500 rad have appeared in only 4 of 24 (17%) of the children tested, as compared to 73 of 95 (77%) of those given doses in excess of 2,500 rad [5]. The follow-up interval is too short to ascertain the impact on gonadal function in prepubertal patients. The use of oophoropexy and appropriate gonadal shielding has allowed the maintenance of menstrual function in girls requiring pelvic irradiation [11]. The ultimate assessment of growth preservation will require many patients and long-term follow-up. However, we are encouraged by a small number of children followed as long as 10 years after low dose irradiation and chemotherapy who show no detectable developmental impairment [18]. There has been no second malignant tumor development among the population receiving low dose irradiation and chemotherapy. However, the median follow-up period in this group is still too short to feel secure, as the median interval from the diagnosis of Hodgkin's disease to the diagnosis of leukemia in the study of *Coleman* et al. [3] was 41 months.

The issue of surgical staging with splenectomy is yet controversial in the pediatric population. The Stanford group has had no complications from operative staging and have greatly reduced the incidence of serious bacterial infections since the routine use of prophylactic antibiotics. The one episode of pneumococcal bacteremia in an asplenic child occurring in the face of antimicrobial prophylaxis occurred in a boy with stage IV Hodgkin's disease involving the bone marrow and liver who was maximally immunosuppressed from 6 cycles of MOPP chemotherapy, and undergoing irradiation at the time of his infection. This occurred 1 year following pneumococcal vaccine injection, 1 year postsplenectomy, and during a time of good compliance to the administration of prophylactic penicillin. Thus, while the use of prophylactic antibiotics has greatly reduced the incidence of serious bacterial infection, there is still a small percentage of children who will develop bacteremia and/or meningitis secondary to encapsulated organisms. Experience with the pneumococcal vaccine suggests that it alone is not sufficient to provide long-term broad protection against the common offending serotypes of the pneumococcus [12]. Whereas others have suggested that an alternative to staging laparotomy with splenectomy is the administration of large volume irradiation and chemotherapy to all children [17], it seems more appropriate to design therapeutic programs in accordance with stage of disease. Irradiation of the spleen is not a nonmorbid alternative to splenectomy, as splenic irradiation is known to produce splenic atrophy and dysfunction capable of resulting in fatal overwhelming sepsis [6]. Furthermore, the accuracy of surgical staging has led the Stanford investigators to decrease the volume of irradiation as well as the dose. The net effect of such treatment is further refinement of therapy and reduction in the known sequelae of irradiation without compromise to the cure rate.

The major hurdle in the treatment of Hodgkin's disease in children is to define the risk/benefit ratio of therapy as it applies to this population with projected long-term survival. It is not possible to directly compare the acute and long-term consequences of a 2–3 months course of radiation against those of a 6-month program of chemotherapy or a 9-month period of combined modality treatment. At the outset it is not possible to predict the impact of altered bone growth, sterility, change in body image, interruption and interference of school and work, or the psychosocial problems related to having a malignant disease. These are the issues which require our attention today and our investigation in the future. At present it appears that the combination of low dose irradiation and chemotherapy is successful in affording optimistic cure rates with minimal morbidity and is therefore appropriate for the majority of children afflicted with Hodgkin's disease.

Acknowledgments

I wish to thank Drs. *H.S. Kaplan, S.A. Rosenberg* and the members of the Lymphoma team at Stanford for their aid in caring for these children, and Miss *Barbara Gilbert* for her secretarial assistance.

References

1 Botnick, L.E.; Goodman, R.; Jaffe, N.; Filler, R.; Cassady, J.R.: Stages I–III Hodgkin's disease in children. Results of staging and treatment. Cancer *39:* 599–603 (1977).

2 Carbone, P.; Kaplan, H.S.; Musshoff, K.; Smithers, D.W.; Tubiana, M.: Report of The Committee on Hodgkin's disease staging classification. Cancer Res. *31:* 1860–1861 (1971).

3 Coleman, C.N.; Williams, C.J.; Flint, A.; Glatstein, E.J.; Rosenberg, S.A.; Kaplan, H.S.: Hematologic neoplasia in patients treated for Hodgkin's disease. New Engl. J. Med. *297:* 1249–1252 (1977).

4 Coltman, C.A.: Chemotherapy of advanced Hodgkin's disease. Semin. in Oncol. *7:* 155–173 (1980).

5 Constine, L.S.; Donaldson, S.S.; McDougall, I.R.; Kaplan, H.S.: Thyroid dysfunction after radiotherapy in children with Hodgkin's disease (Abstract). Int. J. Rad. Oncol. *6:* 1357 (1980).

6 Dailey, M.; Coleman, C.N.; Kaplan, H.S.: Functional asplenia in patients undergoing splenic irradiation. A case report and a review of autopsy cases. New Engl. J. Med. *302:* 217 (1980).

7 DeVita, V.T.; Serpick, A.A.; Carbone, P.P.: Combination chemotherapy in the treatment of advanced Hodgkin's disease. Ann. intern. Med. *73:* 881–895 (1970).

8 Donaldson, S.S.: Pediatric Hodgkin's disease. Focus on the future; in Ed. van Eys, Sullivan; Status of the curability of childhood cancers, pp. 235–249 (Raven Press, New York 1980).

9 Donaldson, S.S.; Glatstein, E.; Kaplan, H.S.: Radiotherapy of childhood lymphoma; in Ed. M.M. Donaldson, Seydel: Trends in childhood cancer, pp. 38–66 (John Wiley, 1976).

10 Donaldson, S.S.; Glatstein, E.; Rosenberg, S.A.; Kaplan, H.S.: Pediatric Hodgkin's disease. II. Results of therapy. Cancer *37:* 2436–2447 (1976).

11 Donaldson, S.S.; Kaplan H.S.: A survey of pediatric Hodgkin's disease at Stanford. Results of therapy and quality of survival; in Ed. Kaplan, Rosenberg, Advances in malignant lymphomas. Etiology, immunology, pathology, and treatment (Academic Press, New York 1982).

12 Donaldson, S.S.; Vosti, K.L.; Berberich, F.R.; Cox, R.S.; Kaplan, H.S.; Schiffman, G.: Response to preumococcal vaccine among children with Hodgkin's disease. Rev. infect. dis. *3:* S133–143 (1981).

13 Gams, R.A.: Complications of chemotherapy in the treatment of Hodgkin's disease. Semin. Oncol. *7:* 184–186 (1980).

14   Hoppe, R.T.: Radiation therapy in the treatment of Hodgkin's disease. Semin. Oncol. *7:* 144–154 (1980).

15   Hoppe, R.T.; Portlock, C.S.; Glatstein, E.; Rosenberg, S.A.; Kaplan, H.S.: Alternating chemotherapy and irradiation in the treatment of advanced Hodgkin's disease. Cancer *43:* 472–481 (1979).

16   Jenkin, D.; Freedman, M.; McClure, P.; Peters, V.; Saunders, F.; Sonley, M.: Hodgkin's disease in children. Treatment with low dose radiation and MOPP without staging laparotomy. A preliminary report. Cancer *44:* 80–86 (1979).

17   Jenkin, R.D.T.; Berry M.P.: Hodgkin's disease in children. Semin. Oncol. *7:* 202–211 (1980).

18   Kaplan, H.S.: Hodgkin's disease; 2nd ed. (Harvard University press, Cambridge 1980).

19   Kaplan, H.S.; Rosenberg, S.A.: The treatment of Hodgkin's disease. Med. Clins. N. Am. *50:* 1591–1610 (1966).

20   Krikorian, J.G.; Burke, J.S.; Rosenberg, S.A.; Kaplan, H.S.: The occurrence of non-Hodgkin's lymphoma following therapy for Hodgkin's disease. New Engl. J. Med. *300:* 452–458 (1979).

21   Olweny, C.L.; Katangole-Mbidde, E.; Kiire, C.; Lwanga, S.K.; Magrath, I.; Ziegler, J.L.: Childhood Hodgkin's disease in Uganda. A ten-year experience. Cancer *42:* 787–792 (1978).

22   Probert, J.C.; Parker, B.R.: The effects of radiation therapy on bone growth. Radiology *114:* 155–162 (1975).

23   Probert, J.C.; Parker, B.R.; Kaplan, H.S.: Growth retardation in children after megavoltage irradiation of the spine. Cancer *32:* 634–639 (1973).

24   Sherins, R.T.; Olweny, C.L.M.; Ziegler, J.L.: Gynecomastia and gonadal dysfunction in adolescent boys treated with combination chemotherapy for Hodgkin's disease. New Engl. J. Med. *299:* 12–16 (1978).

25   Thar, T.L.; Million, R.R.: Complications of radiation treatment of Hodgkin's disease. Semin. Oncol. *7:* 174–183 (1980).

26   Wilimas, J.; Thompson, E.; Smith, K.L.: Long-term results of treatment of children and adolescents with Hodgkin's disease. Cancer *46:* 2123–2125 (1980).

27   Young, R.C.; DeVita, V.T.; Johnson, R.E.: Hodgkin's disease in childhood. Blood *42:* 163–174 (1973).

S.S. Donaldson, MD, Department of Radiology, Division of Radiation Therapy, Stanford University School of Medicine, Stanford, CA 94305 (USA)

Front. Radiat. Ther. Onc., vol. 16, pp. 134–140 (Karger, Basel 1982)

Paediatric Non-Hodgkin's Lymphomas: The Childrens' Cancer Study Group Experience

An Interim Report

R.D.T. Jenkin, J.R. Anderson, R.R. Chilcote, P. Coccia, P. Exelby, J. Kersey, J. Kushner, A. Meadows, S. Siegel, J. Wilson, S. Leiken, D. Hammond

The Children's Cancer Study Group Operations Office, 1721 Griffin Avenue, Los Angeles, Calif. 90031, USA

Introduction

Remarkable improvement has occurred in the cure rate for the childhood non-Hodgkin's lymphomas. Intensive systemic treatment has increased the classical 10–15% cure rate obtained with various local treatment methods to not less than 50–60%. This marked overall improvement was first demonstrated by *Wollner* et al. [6] using the ten drug LSA_2-L_2 regimen. *Wollner* et al. [7] reported equally good results when the disease was predominantly abdominal.

Ziegler [8] demonstrated the effectiveness of cyclophosphamide and methotrexate in North American Burkitt's type lymphoma. Earlier, *Djerassi and Kim* [1] showed the effectiveness of high dose methotrexate in all forms of this disease. *Weinstein and Link* [4] and *Weinstein* et al. [5] used the combination of adriamycin with vincristine, prednisone, *L*-asparaginase and 6 mercaptopurine, although the results with Burkitt's type lymphoma were not satisfactory. *Murphy and Hustu* [3] utilized a cyclophosphamide-intensified leukemic regimen for localized disease and a cyclophosphamide and adriamycin-intensified regimen for more advanced disease, and obtained a 90% disease-free survival rate of 2 years for patients in stages I and II and 39% for stages III and IV. In advanced disease they were not able to demonstrate any benefit from the addition of radiation treatment but obtained suggestive evidence that elective CNS treatment was of value.

Against this background the investigators of CCSG mounted the first large prospective multi-institutional randomized trial, in 1976. They elected to compare two systemic regimens, using on the one hand a modified ten drug LSA_2-L_2 regimen to confirm Wollner's remarkable results and comparing this with a new four drug regimen based on cyclophosphamide and moderately high dose methotrexate. A pilot study with the latter regimen has been reported [2].

In both regimens radiation treatment and CNS prophylaxis were standardized. In localized presentations all known disease was irradiated and in widespread presentations bulk disease was irradiated. CNS prophylaxis was carried out with maintained intrathecal methotrexate. A standard duration of treatment of moderate length, 18 month, was chosen. This study was open to all previously untreated children with any form of non-Hodgkin's lymphoma. An arbitrary distinction from acute leukemia was made by excluding patients with more than 25% blasts in the bone marrow.

The detailed drug dosage schedule is given in table I. During the progress of this study the duration of treatment with cytosine arabinoside and 6-thioguanine during consolidation with the LSA_2-L_2 was reduced from 4 to 2 weeks due to bone marrow toxicity.

Results

Between April 1977 and November 1979, 374 eligible children entered the study and formed the basis of this interim report, an analysis made in December 1980. The overall 3-year survival rate was 66% and the 3-year relapse-free survival rate was 61% (fig. 1). Few adverse events were seen after 2 years. The shape of these curves confirms the findings of all other investigators that the 2-year relapse free rate correlates very closely with the ultimate cure rate. All subsequent data will relate to relapse-free survival rates.

Localized versus Non-Localized Disease
118 patients presented with localized disease, that is with involvement limited to the gastrointestinal tract with or without involved mesenteric nodes; Waldeyer's ring with or without involved cervical nodes; lymph node presentations confined to a single region or two adjacent regions and any of the rare extra-lympatic sites provided that the dis-

Table I. Regimen I (COMP) and regimen II (LSA$_2$-L$_2$), drug dosage and schedule; duration of treatment: 18 months

Induction	Consolidation	Maintenance
Regiment I CMP 1.2 g/m^2, i.v., day 1		1.0 g/m^2, i.v., day 1, repeat q 28 days
VCR 2.0 mg/m^2 (max. 2.0 mg), i.v., weekly on days 3, 10, 17 and 24		1.5 mg/m^2, i.v. (max. dose 2.0 mg), day 1, repeat q 14 days
MTX i.t., 6.25 mg/m^2, day 5 and on days 31 and 34 during PDN withdrawal		i.t., 6.25 mg/m^2, day 29, repeat q 28 days
MTX i.v., 300 mg/m^2 on day 12 (60% of dose as i.v. push and 40% as 4-hour infusion)		i.v., 300 mg/m^2, i.v., day 15, repeat q 28 days (60% of dose i.v. push, 40% as 4 hour infusion)
PDN 60 mg/m^2 (max. 60 mg), p.o. daily, in 4 divided doses, days 3–30, decremental doses to 0, days 31–37 XRT		60 mg/m^2 (max. dose 60 mg), p.o. daily × 5 on day 29, repeat q 28 days
Regimen II CPM 1.2 g/m^2, i.v., day 1	ARA-C 100 mg/m2, i.v., daily × 5 (Monday–Friday) for 4 weeks	cycle: 1 TG-CPM TG, 300 mg/m^2, p.o., daily × 4, followed by CPM, 600 mg/m^2, i.v., single dose, day 5
VCR 2.0 mg/m^2 (max. dose 2.0 mg), i.v., weekly on days 3, 10, 17 and 24	6-TG 50 mg/m^2, p.o., 8–12 h after each ARA-C injection	2 HU-DNM HU, 2.4 g/m^2, p.o., daily × 4, followed by DNM, 45 mg/m^2, i.v. on day 5
MTX 6.25 mg/m^2, i.t., day 5, repeat on days 31 and 34 during PDN withdrawal	*L*-Asp. 6,000 IU/m^2/day × 14, i.m., on completion of ARA-C + 6-TG	3 MTX-BCNU MTX, 10 mg/m^2, p.o., daily × 4, followed by BCNU, 60 mg/m^2, i.v. on day 5
PDN 60 mg/m^2 (max. dose 60 mg), p.o. daily in 4 divided doses, days 3–30, decremental doses to 0, days 31–37	MTX 6.25 mg/m^2, i.t., twice, 3 days apart, begin 2–3 days after last *L*-Asp. injection.	4 ARA-C-VCR ARA-C, 150 mg/m^2, i.v., daily × 4, followed by CVR 2.0 mg/m^2 (max. dose 2.0 mg) i.v. day 5
DNM 60 mg/m^2, i.v., days 12 and 13	BCNU 60 mg/m^2, i.v., single dose 2–3 days following completion of i.t. MTX	5 MTX 6.25 mg/m^2, i.t., 2 doses, 3 days apart.

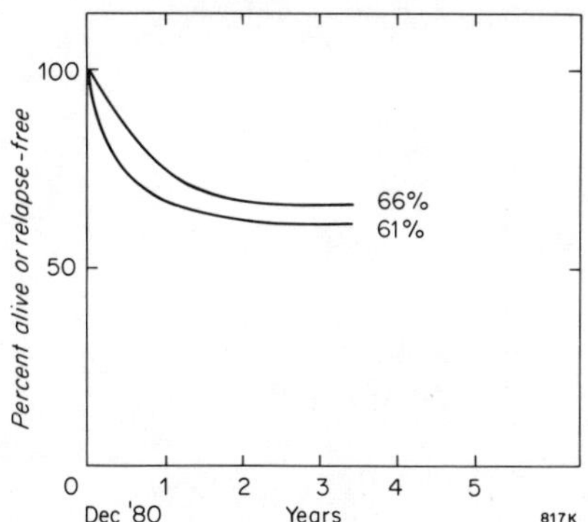

Fig. 1. CCG-551. Survival and relapse-free survival. All patients.

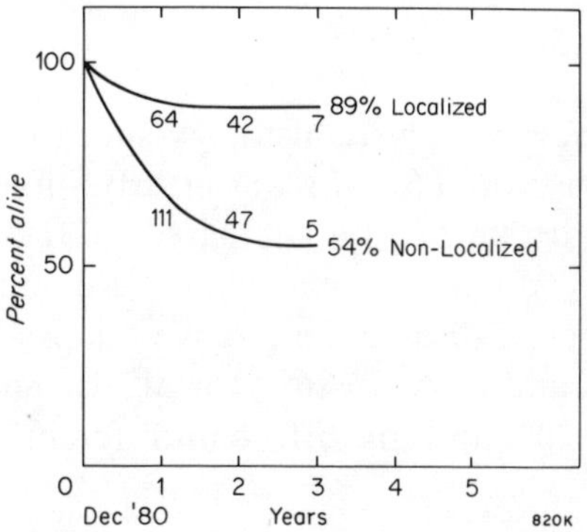

Fig. 2. Survival for patients with localized (n = 118) and non-localized (n = 256) disease at diagnosis.

ease was limited to a single site with or without involved regional nodes. Mediastinal mass presentations were specifically excluded and classified as non-localized; the 3-year relapse-free survival rate was 89% (fig. 2). Conversely, 256 patients presented with non-localized disease; the 3-year relapse-free survival rate was 54% (fig. 2).

LSA$_2$-L$_2$ versus COMP

Overall there was no difference in 3-year relapse-free survival rates by regimen: LSA$_2$-L$_2$ 60% and COMP 57%. In localized disease the two regimens were also equally effective with 3-year relapse-free rates: LSA$_2$-L$_2$ 81% and COMP 85%.

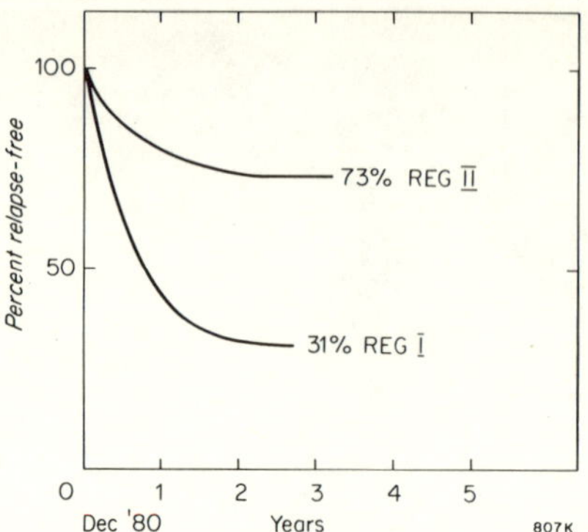

Fig. 3. Relapse-free survival for patients with non-localized lymphoblastic disease by treatment regimen. Regimen I (n = 28) = COMP; regimen II (n = 33) = LSA₂-L₂. p = 0.005.

In non-localized disease the regimens were histology-specific. For patients with lymphoblastic disease the LSA₂-L₂ was clearly superior with a 3-year relapse-free survival rate of 73% compared to 31% for COMP (fig. 3). The converse was true for patients with non-lymphoblastic disease: For diffuse histiocytic disease the relative relapse-free rates at 2 years were COMP 69% and LSA₂-L₂ 26%; for diffuse undifferentiated Burkitt's type 64 and 20% and for diffuse undifferentiated pelomorphic type 59 and 29%.

Discussion

To date, this study has confirmed that a modified LSA₂-L₂ treatment will produce improved results in children with non-Hodgkin's lymphoma and has demostrated that similar overall results may be obtained with a four drug programme, COMP. The important observation is that each of these regimens for non-localized disease is histology-specific with COMP superior for non-lymphoblastic disease and LSA₂-L₂ superior for lymphoblastic disease.

In patients with localized disease it appears that both systemic treatments are effective. Allowing for approximately a 5% toxic death rate in remission both regimens can eradicate non-Hodgkin's lymphoma when the body burden of tumour cells is relatively small with an effectiveness of about 90%. About one-third of these patients present with localized disease and in approximately 80% of these patients the histology is non-lymphoblastic. Thus, in this study very few patients with localized lymphoblastic disease were treated with COMP and for that reason larger numbers must be available for this sub-set, before, there can be any certainty that COMP is an adequate treatment.

The duration of treatment, 18 months, appeared adequate at least in that relapse after 2 years was very uncommon. The optimal duration of treatment is clearly the minimum duration that will maintain the reported results. This duration is not known.

Since no question was asked in this study regarding radiation therapy no answer will emerge. In patients with localized disease a first relapse in the irradiated volume was not seen in this study. It can thus be stated that for these patients when effective systemic treatment is given the irradiation dose should not exceed 3,000 rad in 15–20 fractions for local volumes or 2,000 rad in 20 fractions for the whole abdomen. Optimal doses may be lower. The effectiveness of a policy of radiation for sites of bulk disease in non-localized patients cannot be assessed in this study, although it was clear that relapse in the irradiated volumes was exceptionally uncommon.

The incidence of an isolated first relapse in the CNS was low in this study at 7%, which circumstantially would suggest that there was at least a very large sub-set for whom this treatment was necessary.

This first large study of unselected children with non-Hodgkin's lymphoma has confirmed that the majority of these children can be cured. Optimal treatment with current agents remains to be determined. The major difference observed in this study between the regimens in patients with non-localized disease indicated that we can anticipate a 70% cure rate when the appropriate histology specific regimen is utilized.

References

1   Djerassi, I.; Kim, J.S.: Methotrexate and citrovorum factor rescue in the management of childhood lymphosarcoma and reticulum cell sarcoma (non-Hodgkin's lymphomas). Cancer *38:* 1043–1051 (1976).

2   Meadows, A.T.; Jenkin, R.D.T.; Anderson, J.P.; Chilcote, R.; Coccia, P.; Exelby, P.; Kushner, J.; Leikin, S.; Siegel, S.; Wilson, J.S.; Hammond, D.: A new therapy schedule for pediatric non-Hodgkin's lymphoma: toxicity and preliminary research. Med. Pediat. Oncol. *8:* 15–24 (1980).

3   Murphy, S.B.; Hustu, H.O.: A randomized trial of combined modality therapy of childhood non-Hodgkin's lymphoma. Cancer 45:630–637 (1980).
4   Weinstein, H.J.; Link, M.P.: Non-Hodgkin's lymphoma in childhood Clin. Haematol. 8:699–716 (1979).
5   Weinstein, H.; Vance, Z,; Jaffe, N.; Buell, D.; Cassady, J.; Nathan, D: Improved prognosis for patients with mediastinal lymphoblastic lymphoma. Blood 53: 687–694 (1979).
6   Wollner, N.; Exelby, P.R.; Lieberman, P.H.: Non-Hodgkin's lymphoma in children. Cancer 44:1990–1999 (1979).
7   Wollner, N.; Wachtel, A.E.; Exelby, P.R.; Centore, D.: Improved prognosis in children with intra-abdominal non-Hodgkin's lymphoma following LSA_2-L_2 protocol chemotherapy. Cancer 45:3034–3039 (1980.
8   Ziegler, J.L.: Treatment results of fifty-four American patients with Burkitt's lymphoma are similat to the African experience. New Engl. Med. 297:75–80 (1977).

R.D.T. Jenkin, MB, Professor of Radiology, University of Toronto, The Ontario Cancer Foundation, Toronto-Bayview Clinic, 2075 Bayview Avenue, Toronto, Ont. M4N 3M5 (Canada)

Front. Radiat. Ther. Onc., vol. 16, pp. 141–149 (Karger, Basel 1982)

Malignant Germ Cell Tumors in Children[1]

Arthur R. Ablin

Division of Pediatric Hematology and Oncology, University of California,
San Francisco, Calif., USA

Introduction

My goals will be to (1) demonstrate the interrelationship of germ cell tumors of differing histologies and various sites; (2) to review the significance of the biochemical markers characteristic of some germ cell tumors, and (3) to update the current therapy and prognosis of germ cell tumors.

Embryology

Primordial germ cells most probably originate in the yolk sac endoderm and find their way into the developing fetus, probably by the 5th or 6th week of fetal life, through the dorsal mesentery of the hind gut and thence to the urogenital ridge (fig. 1). This ridge, which subsequently separates into medial genital and a lateral mesonephric structure, extends in the fetus cephalocaudad from C6 to S2. Their path from yolk sac to gonads is at times a meandering and devious one and primordial germinal tissue finds itself in strange places. When these cells or their progeny undergo malignant transformation, tumors occur either in gonadal sites for those cells which have hit their mark or extragonadal tumors for those which have erred (table I).

[1] This investigation was supported by PHS grant No. CA 17829 awarded by the National Cancer Institute, DHHS.

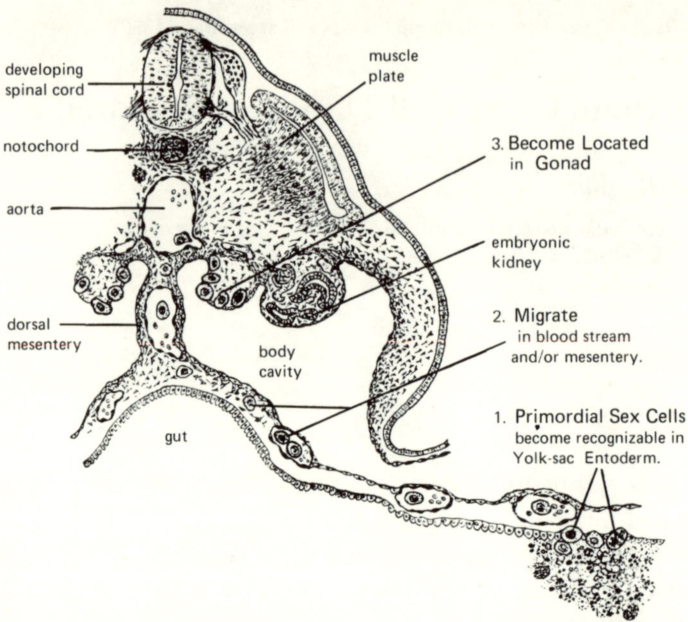

Fig. 1. Schema depicting the migration of totapotential germ cells from yolk sac to gonad (from *Patten's* Human Embryology).

Table I. Sites of germ cell tumors

Gonadal
Ovarian
Testicular
Extragonadal
Sacrococcygeal
Intracranial (pituitary, pineal, cerebellar, other)
Anterior mediastinal
Retroperitoneal
MSC (thymus, orbit, parotid, naso-pharynx, umbilical, neck, tonsil)

Pathological Classification

The classification of germ cell tumors advanced by *Teilum* [21] is now widely accepted and provides an excellent explanation of the interrelationship of these tumors (fig. 2). Primordial germ cells can replicate and produce other undifferentiated primordial cells or differ-

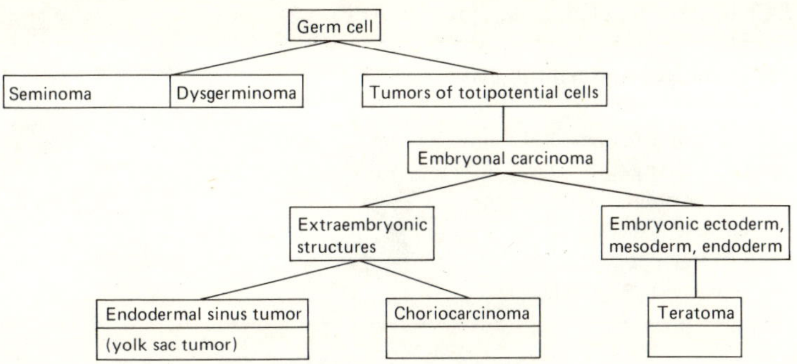

Fig. 2. Teilum's [21] classification of germ cell tumors.

entiate prior to further replication. Both of these processes occur with greater frequency in the male gonad than the female and this most probably accounts for the greater frequency of testicular tumors when compared with ovarian. When the primordial germ cell finds its mark in the ovary or testis and has very little differentiation but undergoes malignant transformation, it produces a monophasic tumor in the ovary called a dysgerminoma and an identical tumor in the testis, a seminoma. These same tumors in extragonadal sites are germinomas. When some differentiation of the primordial germ cells occurs after which a malignant transformation occurs, an epithelial tumor composed of solid sheets of large polygonal or ovoid cells containing primitive epithelium appears, which is called an embryonal carcinoma. If, however, further differentiation takes place before the transforming event, uncontrolled replication can lead to tumors which are histologically similar to embryonic or extraembryonic structures. Those extraembryonic structures can resemble gestational tissues and when mixtures of syncytiotrophoblastic cytotrophoblastic tissues occur, the tumor produced is a choriocarcinoma. When the extraembryonic structures resemble the endodermal sinus in the mouse placenta, they may be called yolk sac or endodermal sinus tumors. When differentiation of germ cells results in the formation of embryonic ectoderm, mesoderm, or endoderm, and all three of these elements are found together in one tissue mass, they are teratomas. When these elements show evidence of malignant transformation they are malignant teratomas, and otherwise are benign. One can readily understand how in a single tumor varying degrees of differentiation have occurred before uncontrolled replica-

Table II. Characteristics of alpha-fetoprotein (AFP)

Glycoprotein, molecular weight 70,000
Normally produced in fetus:
   Yolk sac, liver, gastrointestinal tract
   12th week 3×10^6 ng/ml
   Predominant protein
Metabolic half-life: 5 days
Normal value after 1 year < 16 ng/ml
Sensitivity of assay: 1–5 ng/ml

tion starts, and one could therefore expect to find germ cell tumors of mixed histology.

Tumor Markers

As might be expected, these primitive cells are capable of producing significant biochemical markers which have proven to be clinically important in diagnosis and establishing prognosis.

Alpha-Fetoprotein

It has been known for many years that the developing fetus contains a protein which is absent or present in only trace amounts in the adult [3]. In the fetus, this counterpart to adult albumin is called alpha-fetoprotein. In 1967, *Abelev* [1] described the presence of alpha-fetoprotein in the serum of adults with teratocarcinoma of the ovary and testis. Shortly thereafter, *Gitlin* et al. [8] demonstrated that alpha-fetoprotein was synthesized in the human yolk sac. Some characteristics of alpha-fetoprotein are listed in table II.

Human Chorionic Gonadotropin

Specialized placental cells are capable of producing a glycoprotein with a molecular weight of 38,000 which is related to continuing successful implantation of the fertilized egg and a proper maternal-fetal relationship. This protein is composed of two polypeptide chains, alpha and beta, which chemically resemble the structure of pituitary-luteinizing hormone, thyrotropic hormone, and follicle-stimulating hormone. However, the beta subunit can be immunologically separated

Table III. Characteristics of human chorionic gonadotropin (hCG)

Glycoprotein: molecular weight 38,000
Produced by specialized placental cells
Composed of 2 polypeptide chains: alpha and beta
Resembles chemical structure of pituitary LH, TH, FSH
RIA separates beta subunit of placental hCG from
    pituitary LH, TH, FSH
Half-life: whole molecule 30 h, beta subunit 45 min
Sensitivity of beta subunit assay: <1 ng/ml

from its chemically similar beta chain on the pituitary hormones. With the development of this radioimmunoassay it is possible to distinguish chorionic gonadotropin of nonpituitary origin from the pituitary hormones (table III). Thus, tumor production can be monitored.

Those tumors which contain placental or gestational elements can be expected to produce chorionic gonadotropin. Germ cell tumors which contain choriocarcinoma or germinomas with trophoblastic differentiation produce choriocarcinoma. Other conditions in which human chorionic gonadotropin (hCG) is elevated are liver, breast, stomach, pancreatic and lung tumors. Of course, gestational trophoblastic disease, such as hydatiform moles, is another producer of this glycoprotein as is certainly the luxurient growth of placental tissue in normal pregnancy.

Clinical Characteristics

Seminomas spread through the regional lymph nodes and only late and relatively rarely develop hematogenous metastasis. Since these tumors are relatively radiosensitive, local excision with lymphadenectomy or nodal radiation is predictably curable. Most other germ cells spread both via the lymphatics and by the blood stream, and therapy aimed at cure must consider both of these routes of spread. Special consideration is due the yolk sac tumor in children under 2 years of age where lymphatic spread is unusual and hematogenous spread is more likely to occur than in its counterpart, embryonal carcinoma in the older male. Orchiectomy alone may be satisfactory in children under 2 years of age provided hormonal markers which were positive prior to surgery return to negative postoperatively. Chemotherapy with or without lymphadenectomy, however, would be recommended if there is not a drop in the markers to normal limits in a time period consistent with the known half-life of the marker.

The Evolution of Treatment and Results

Prior to 1950 there was no effective therapy for malignant germ cell tumors and only some of those who could be completely resected survived the disease. These were rare and fortunate patients. In 1956 *Li* et al. [14] made observations while working with folic acid antagonists and mice. They noted that hypophysectomized mice with metastatic melanoma dropped their hCG to zero when treated with amethopterin. They reasoned that hCG-producing tumors might respond to the same drug. This resulted in the treatment of gestational choriocarcinoma with methotrexate with a 47% complete response (CR). Unfortunately, nongestational choriocarcinoma was not responsive to methotrexate and remains today the most dificult of germ cells to treat. In 1960, *Li* et al. [15] reported that disseminated testicular germ cells had a 20% CR rate to combination methotrexate, chlorambucil, and actinomycin. Other reports in the 60s report 5–10% survival with surgery, radiation therapy and various single and combination agent chemotherapy. In the first half of the 70s, several single agents were found to produce significant response rates in disseminated testicular germ cell tumor. *Kennedy* [13] reported a 37% CR + partial response (PR) with methramycin but also major toxic effects. *Samuels and Howe* [16] reported a 52% CR + PR with velban. *Blum* et al. [4] reviewed the use of bleomycin and reported a 32% CR + PR. *Higby* et al. [11] reported a 28% CR with the use of cisplatinum. *Samuels* et al. [17] combined velban and bleomycin postulating that velban arrested cells in mitosis and bleomycin was effective on mitotic cells as well as cells which were synchronized to enter the phase of DNA synthesis. The 70s saw the Memorial Group in New York City producing a succession of VAB (velban, actinomycin and bleomycin) protocols. This combination produced only a 22% CR when reported in 1973 [19]. *Samuels* et al. [18], taking note of earlier reported improved effectiveness of bleomycin when given continuously rather than intermittently, produced a 53% complete remission rate with velban continuous bleomycin. *Einhorn and Donohue* [6] in Indiana, drawing on this previous combined velban, bleomycin and platinum, produced an astounding 70% complete remission rate in disseminated testicular tumors. When platinum and continuous bleomycin were added to VAB-I, i.e. VAB-II [5], the remission rate went up to 58%. In 1976, *Wolner* et al. [23] reported a small group of children with ovarian tumors who had a 60% survival when treated with a combination of vincristine, actinomycin, cytoxan, and adriamycin. When adriamycin was added in the PVB regimen, *Einhorn and Donohue* [7] reported a 100% CR + PR.

Both the Indiana and Memorial Groups realized when their data was analyzed that many of their CR patients were relapsing, and the relapse rate seemed to be independent of the maintenance therapy. It became evident that it was important to give more intensive therapy early in the treatment of patients with disseminated germ cell tumor and that long maintenance therapy might not be beneficial. It was known that platinum was an effective drug for germ cell tumors, but the amount of platinum that could be administered was seriously limited by its renal toxicity. The Memorial Group [10] demonstrated in 1977 with animal and human work that it was safe to give larger doses of platinum, 100–120 mg/m², if maximum diuresis was achieved at the time the platinum was given. This allowed for the development of the VAB-III protocol when a high dose of platinum was combined with bleomycin, cytoxan and chlorambucil and a 62% CR resulted. When early treatment was intensified in VAB-III and VAB-IV the complete remission rate went up to 73 and 92%, respectively [9]. The most recent development was in the Indiana Group [22] when refractory disseminated germ cell tumors were found to be responsive to the epipodophyllotoxin preparation VP 16 when it was combined with platinum, bleomycin and adriamycin even in patients who had previously been unresponsive to the later agents.

The Children's Cancer Group in a recently developed and ongoing study for the treatment of germ cell tumors in children, excluding testicular tumors, has used the drug combination successful in adult testicular tumors developed in Indiana, New York, and Houston, namely velban, bleomycin and platinum, and combined those agents with previously effective drugs, actinomycin, adriamycin and cytoxan. Children are treated for 18 weeks at which time second-look surgery for all children is performed. Those that are tumor-free continue with the same chemotherapy for a total of 102 weeks while those that are found to have tumor present at second surgery receive radiation therapy prior to continuing chemotherapy. The study is too early to evaluate but thus far 12 nonovarian tumors have been treated, 8 of which have no evidence of disease, either proven at surgery [5] or by being followed with markers and diagnostic imagery [3]. 1 patient had a PR and 3 patients are in treatment and it is too early to evaluate them. 2 of the patients have died, 1 a CR and 1 a PR patient. Of the ovarian tumors, there were 17 eligible patients, 13 of which achieved CR status, 2 patients had partial remission, and 2 patients were not in therapy long enough to evaluate. 3 patients, however, died. 2 of these patients had ruptured tumors at the time of diagnosis but achieved complete remission before progression. 1 patient with metastatic disease achieved a good partial remission prior to recurrence and death. In our series all patients achieved either a CR or PR.

We acknowledge the important influence that the therapy of disseminated adult germ cell tumors has had on the therapy of children with histologically similar disease. There has been steady progress since the 50s, 60s and 70s. There is no question that many young children with germ cell tumors who would have died in the 60s, will be alive in the 80s and the era of the 80s is expected to see 80–90% of the individuals with malignant germ cell tumors surviving – an appropriate ending for a discussion of malignant germ cell tumors in this Symposium on 'Triumph over Tragedy'.

References

1   Abelev, G.I.: Embryonal serum alpha globulin in cancer patients. Int. J. Cancer *2:* 551 (1967).
2   Abell, M.R.; Johnson, V.J.; Holtz, F.: Ovarian neoplasms in childhood and adolescence. Am. J. Obstet Gynec. *92:* 1059 (1965).
3   Bergstrand, C.G.; Czar, B.: Demonstration of a new protein fraction in serum from a human fetus. Scand. J. clin. Lab. Invest. *8:* 174 (1956).
4   Blum, R.H.; Carter, S.; Agre, K.: A clinical review of bleomycin – a new antineoplastic agent. Cancer *31:* 903 (1973).
5   Cvitkovic, E.; Wittes, R.; Golbey, R.B. et al.: Primary combination chemotherapy (VAB II) for metastatic unresectable germ cell tumors. Proc. Am. Ass. Cancer Res. *16:* 695 (1975).
6   Einhorn, L.H.; Donohue, J.P.: Cis-diaminodichloroplatinum, vinblastine and bleomycin combination chemotherapy in disseminated testicular cancer. Ann. intern. Med. *87:* 293 (1977).
7   Einhorn, L.H.; Donohue, J.P.: Combination chemotherapy in disseminated testicular cancer. Seminars in Oncol. *6:* 87 (1979).

8   Gitlin, D.; Pericelli, A.; Gitlin, G.M.: Synthesis of fetoprotein by liver, yolk sac and gastrointestinal tract of the human conceptus. Cancer Res. *32:*979 (1972).
9   Golbey, R.B.; Reynolds, T.F.; Vugrin, D.: Chemotherapy of metastatic germ cell tumors. Semin. Oncol. *6:*82 (1979).
10 Hayes, D.M.; Cvitkovic, E.; Golbey, R. et al.: High dose cisplatinum diamine dichloride. Amelioration of renal toxicity by mannitol diuresis. Cancer *39:* 1371 (1977).
11 Higby, D.J.; Wallace, H.J.; Albert, D., et al.: Diaminodichloro-platinum in chemotherapy of testicular tumors. J. Urol. *112:*100 (1974).
12 Huntington, R.W.; Bullock, W.K.: Yolk sac tumors of the ovary. Cancer *25:* 1357 (1970).
13 Kennedy, B.J.: Mithramycin therapy in advanced testicular neoplasms. Cancer *26:* 755 (1970).
14 Li, M.C.; Hertz, R.; Spencer, D.B.: Effect of methotrexate therapy upon choriocarcinoma and chorioadenoma. Proc. Soc. exp. Biol. Med. *96:*361 (1956).
15 Li, M.C.; Whitmore, W.F.; Golbey, R.B., et al.: Effects of combined drug therapy in treatment of testicular tumors. J. Am. med. Ass. *174:*245 (1960).
16 Samuels, M.L.; Howe, C.D.: Vinblastine in the management of testicular cancer. Cancer *25:*1009 (1970).
17 Samuels, M.L.; Johnson, D.E.; Holoye, P.Y.: The treatment of stage 3 metastatic germinal neoplasia of the testis with bleomycin combination therapy. Proc. Am. Ass. Cancer Res. *14:*89 (1973).
18 Samuels, M.L.; Johnson, D.E.; Holoye, P.Y.: Continuous intravenous bleomycin therapy with vinblastine in stage III testicular neoplasia. Cancer Chemother. Rep. *59:*563 (1975).
19 Silway, O.; Yagoda, A.; Wittes, R., et al.: Treatment of germ cell carcinomas with a combination of actinomycin D, vinblastine and bleomycin. Proc. Am. Ass. Cancer Res. *14:*271 (1973).
20 Smith, J.P.; Rutledge, F.: Advances in chemotherapy for gynecologic cancer. Cancer *36:*669 (1975).
21 Teilum, G.: Classification of endodermal sinus tumor (meioblastoma vitellinum) and so-called embryonal carcinoma of the ovary. Acta path. microbiol. scand. *64:* 407 (1965).
22 Williams, S.O.; Einhorn, L.H.; Greco, A., et al.: VP-16-213 salvage therapy for refractory germinal neoplasms. Cancer *46:*2154 (1980).
23 Wolner, N.; Exelby, P.; Woodruff, J.M., et al.: Malignant ovarian tumors in childhood. Prognosis in relation to initial therapy. Cancer *37:*1953 (1976).

A.R. Ablin, MD, Department of Pediatrics – M650, University of California School of Medicine, San Francisco, CA 94143 (USA)

Front. Radiat. Ther. Onc., vol. 16, pp. 150–152 (Karger, Basel 1982)

Histiocytosis X

Joseph H. Kushner

University of California, San Francisco, Calif., USA

Histiocytosis is a complex group of disorders ranging from only one or several bones being involved with small osteolytic lesions [1, 13, 14] (causing no disability and responding rapidly to either curetting or low-dose x-ray therapy [2] to very severe systemic disease with organ dysfunction and malignant histology with almost always a fatal outcome [5, 11].

To further subdivide this group into prognostic groups [3] is to determine [1] whether or not organ dysfunction exists [4], and [2] whether it is 'benign' or 'malignant' histology [7]. Initial workup should include a bone survey [9], bone scan, liver/spleen scan, chest x-ray, and CT of any involved areas to further delineate the extent of the involvement [1, 8, 10].

More detailed studies of hematopoietic function with bone marrow aspiration and/or biopsy and repeated CBCs and platelet counts evaluate this organ system.

The liver is evaluated with liver function tests, i.e. the presence of hypoproteinemia less than 5.5 g%, the presence of ascites, hyperbilirubinemia, prolonged prothrombin or PTT [4].

Lung organ dysfunction includes any evidence of tachypnea, dyspnea, cyanosis, pneumothorax or pleural effusion [4]. Lung dysfunction does *not* include nodular or cystic lung lesions by x-ray. Pulmonary function studies, of course, form a baseline for any change of lung function.

Careful histologic [6] appearance of the 'benign' lesions includes histiocytes predominating, exhibiting a syncytial appearance, with indistinct cell membranes, polygonal-shaped cells, fibrosis in some areas, focal necrosis and hemorrhage in others; hemosiderin granules, multinuclear giant cells with Langerhans' granules [1], and x-bodies designate a 'benign' lesion on electron microscopy.

A 'malignant' lesion is characterized by a diffuse infiltrate of individual histiocytes throughout the reticuloendothelial system. These histiocytes are large, with abundant weakly basophilic cytoplasm and distinct cell membranes. Nuclei are folded, and the chromatin is clumped. Multinuclear giant cells, eosinophils, necrosis or fibrosis are only rarely seen[7].

A careful immunological workup is also indicated with an x-ray of the thymus, quantitative immunoglobulins hemagglutinins, B and T lymphocyte studies, phytohemagglutinin stimulation, with lymphocyte blastogenesis, karyotyping, and MLC between mother and patient, because of the possibility of graft versus host reaction or immunodeficiency resembling histiocytosis. It is of interest that on autopsy of fatal cases of this disease, thymic dysplasia has been seen in well over two-thirds of those cases in which it has been looked for [13]. Over half of the cases have elevation of immunoglobulin M. All of the above suggests an immunodeficiency disease in the more severe cases. Chemotherapy of the more severe cases consists of four drugs for the 12-week *induction* therapy, including prednisone 40 mg/m²/day on day 1–42, tapered over the next 2-week period. Velban is given 6.5 mg/m² weekly for 12 weeks increasing to 7.0 mg/m² and 7.5 mg/m² if the granulocyte count remains over 1,000. Methotrexate at 10 mg/m²/week orally for 12 weeks and Cytoxan 100 mg/m² weekly by mouth for 12 weeks. The Velban is given on day 1 of each cycle, methotrexate day 2, and Cytoxan on day 4 [3].

Maintenance therapy consists of 6-mercaptopurine 50 mg/m² daily orally for 6 months, methotrexate 10 mg/m² orally on day 1 of each week for 6 months, and Cytoxan 100 mg/m² orally on day 4 of each week for 6 months. If the patient tolerates the above doses for 4 weeks, the methotrexate and Cytoxan are increased every 2 weeks toward the maximum dose of 20 mg/m² of methotrexate and 200 mg/m² of Cytoxan, keeping the poly count (also called absolute neutrophil count) above 1,000 and the platelets in excess of 100,000. If the platelet count drops below 50,000 on the poly count below 1,000, chemotherapy is discontinued, then restarted at a lower dose [3].

Sequelae such as diabetes insipidus, small stature, chronic active histiocytic disease, exophthalmos, tooth loss, skull deformity, vertebral compression, or pulmonary fibrosis and compromise of pulmonary function often occur.

Well over half of the advanced disease patients achieve a complete response with four-drug therapy. Another quarter have a partial response [3]. However, there is still considerable mortality in the advanced disease [Letterer-Siwe; 5, 11] group, and further subclassifications and modifications of therapy will have to be done to achieve an even better result than that which can be obtained at this time.

References

1   Geiser, C.F.: The histiocytosis syndromes. Pediat. Ann. *8:*54–64 (1979).
2   Greenberger, J.S.; Cassady, J.R.; Jaffe, N.; Vawter, G.; Crocker, A.C.: Radiation therapy in patients with histiocytosis: management of diabetes insipidus and bone lesions. Int. J. Radiat. Oncol. Biol. Phys. *5:*1749–1755 (1979).
3   Lahey, M.E.: Histiocytosis X. Comparison of three treatment regimens. J. Pediat. *87:*179–189 (1975).
4   Lahey, M.E.; Heyn, R.M.; Newton, W.A., Jr.; Shore, N.; Smith, W.B.; Leikin, S.; Hammond, D.: Histiocytosis X: clinical trial of chlorambucil: a report from Children's Cancer Study Group. Med. Pediat. Oncol. *7:*197–203 (1979).
5   Letterer, E.: Aleukämische Retikulosis. Z. Path. *30:*377 (1924).
6   Lichtenstein, L.: Histiocystosis X, integration of eosinophilic granuloma of bone, Letterer-Siwe disease, and 'Schuller-Christian disease' as related manifestations of a single nosological entity. Archs. Path. *50:*84–102 (1953).
7   Newton, W.A.; Hamoudi, A.B.: Histiocytosis: a histologic classification with clinical correlation. Perspect. pediatr. Pathol. Yb. *1973:*251–283.
8   Nezelof, C.; Frileux-Herbet, F.; Cronier-Sachot, J.: Disseminated histiocytosis X: analysis of prognostic factors based on a retrospective study of 50 cases. Cancer *44:* 1824–1838 (1979).
9   Parker, B.R.; Pinckney, L.; Etcubanas, E.: Relative efficacy of radiographic and radionuclide bone surveys in the detection of the skeletal lesions of histiocytosis X[1]. Radiology *134:*377–380 (1980).
10 Scully, R.E.; Galdabini, J.J.; McNeely, B.U.: Case records of the Massachusetts General Hospital. New Engl. J. Med. *302:*456–460 (1980).
11 Siwe, S.A.: Die Reticuloendotheliose: ein neues Krankheitsbild unter den Hepatosplenomegalien. Z. Kinderheilk. *55:*212 (1933).
12 Starling, K.A.; Iyer, R.; Silva-Sossa, M.; Komp, D.; Herson, J.; Trueworthy, R.C.: Chlorambucil in histiocytosis X: a Southwest Oncology Group study. J. Pediat. *96:* 266–268 (1980).
13 Williams, J.W.; Dorfman, R.F.: Lymphadenopathy as the initial manifestation of histiocytosis X. Am. J. surg. Pathol. *3:*405–421 (1979).
14 Zucker, J.M.; Caillaux, J.M.; Vanel, D.; Gerard-Marchant, R.: Malignant histiocytosis in childhood: clinical study and therapeutic results in 22 cases. Cancer *45:* 2821–2829 (1980).

Prof. J.H. Kushner, MD, University of California, San Francisco, CA 94143 (USA)

Front. Radiat. Ther. Onc., vol. 16, pp. 153–155 (Karger, Basel 1982)

Discussion

Audience: Dr. *Ablin,* how do you use the hormone markers in terms of response to chemotherapy? Do you see this as a tool that you could utilize to more selectively use the drugs, maybe smaller numbers of drugs or a less toxic regimen?

Ablin: The hormone markers that I talked about, HCG and alpha-fetoprotein, have proven to be extremely reliable. When the tumor is completely resected or when the malignant components of a tumor are gone and only the mature elements, for example, in mature benign keratoma, remain, the markers return to zero. We have noticed that when our patients have died, in every instance with recurrence of tumor the markers have returned. All the CR patients had absence of markers, and with recurrence of disease the markers have appeared. Specifically, the answer to your question is 'Yes, we use the markers'. I believe children under two who have embryonal carcinoma of the testes and whose alpha-fetoprotein drops to zero, don't need any chemotherapy after orchiectomy. It is a very valuable adjunct.

Audience: Do you find this of any use in prognosis in terms of response of a disease?

Ablin: Our 2 partial remission patients and many others reported in the literature failed to have absence of markers, and on recurrence of their disease, their alpha-fetoprotein increased. Yes, they are very reliable.

Audience: Other than the thymic hormone, has any form of immunotherapy been used in soft tissue sarcomas, e.g. vaccines?

Kushner: I don't know, but there has been an excellent symposium on new forms of immunotherapy. Interferon, of course, is the one that we're all watching with a great deal of interest.

Donaldson: The Stanford Interferon data is with a subset of non-Hodgkin's lymphoma patients, and I'm not aware of any data on vaccines in pediatric malignancies.

Audience: I think it's well to know that bacterial vaccines produce endogenous interferon and that they have been used in quite large numbers of osteogenic sarcomas and soft tissue sarcomas producing as high as 80% 5-year survival if they were given for at least 6 months.

Schroeder: Dr. *Donaldson,* what ist the time and dose relationship on low dose or modified dose? What size fractions and over what period of time and total dose?

Donaldson: We're using 1,500 rad for children with a bone age of 6 or less, 2,000 rad for the children that fall in the group of bone age 7–10, and 2,500 rad for the children with bone age of 11–14. Patients over the age of 14 go onto or adult protocol. The volumes are determined by the pathologic staging. The fractionation of radiation really depends on what the volume is, but it's usually 200 rad treating 5 times a week.

Audience: One of the other problems in growth of these children who are irradiated aside from sitting height is a narrow neck, and the short interscapular distances. Have you noticed that your lower doses that you are using now produce less deformity of this kind?

Donaldson: The children that have received low dose radiation all look normal, and we are gratified by that. We have not seen the clavicular shortening in that segment of patients as compared to those patients that get that abnormality with 4,400 rad. But we have only a small number of patients. Although we have treated 48 patients, the median is still 3 years. I'm hesitant to say very much about the long-term bone growth effects from the low dose radiation and MOPP.

Jenkin: There is no doubt that the lower the dose the less the defect. We have used lower doses of about the same size as Dr. *Donaldson* for a few years. Before that we used a lower dose than the Stanford 3,500 rad in 20 fractions, and with that dose one certainly saw late effects, particularly if the child was young at the time of treatment.

Ablin: The problem of second malignant neoplasms in irradiated Hodkin's disease patients with multiple agent chemotherapy is, of course, of great concern. There is an observation made by the Milan group reported about a year ago in the British medical literature that patients, adults as well as children, who were treated with ABVD as well as with radiation therapy had no leukemias, non-Hodgkin's lymphoma or solid tumors. It is of interest that ABVD includes adriamycin, and the late effect study group seems to have identified that actiomycin at least appears to decrease the risk of second malignant neoplasms. It raises the possibility that adriamycin, which is so similar to actinomycin in many of its molecular and clinical effects, may be acting in a similar protective fashion. The interesting corollary piece of evidence is that patients treated with MABOP, which also includes adriamycin, did get second malignant neoplasms. This suggests that adriamycin may protect against radiation associated tumors but not those that are associated with alkylating agents. The future insofar as combined chemo and radiation therapy is concerned is an interesting one, possibly with the consideration of the protective effect of the antibiotics.

Jenkin: If one considers the Stanford and Toronto studies of about 100 children, nearly all of whom are surviving over the last 7 or 8 years, there is not yet an example of a second tumor.

Kushner: We've learned about the azospermia of MOPP therapy, we know about the azospermia of cytoxan therapy. Does anyone have any experience with the various other chemotherapeutic agents we use for ALL?

Audience: A long-term surveillance study is being done at the M.D. Anderson Hospital. Sperm counts of about 20 or 25 younger patients have been analyzed. It would appear that the majority of leukemic patients have no problems as far as spermatogenesis is concerned. The patients in whom abnormalities were detected were principally those in whom radiation seemed to have had an effect on the testes in one way or another, e.g. in treatment of Hodgkin's disease. While it is a little discouraging to note that of the Stanford series 6 patients who were treated with MOPP did not have spermatogenesis (and apparently they were treated in the postpubertal period). There is a study from the NCI in which the sperm counts were evaluated at various times after discontinuation of MOPP chemotherapy. While, indeed, some patient did not have an adequate number of sperm, they subsequently had regeneration of the sperm. It may not necessarily be a permanent feature, and, in fact, some of these patients also later fathered children. While the outlook may initially appear bleak, it may not eventually turn out to be so.

Audience: We are concentrating on sterility, but in the MOPP-treated male there is a hormonal aspect as well. In the Uganda study of patients who were adolescent at the time they received MOPP, those patients were essentially made euniuchoid and devel-

oped gynecomastia as well as aspermia. The younger patients were not so effected insofar as their hormonal status was concerned. In another study by the NCI group in girls, a
similar sort of observation was made. In leukemic girls treated with multiple agent chemotherapy, if they were treated at the time they were menarcheal, then they became more
effected insofar as ovarian function is concerned than younger girls or those who were
well established postadolescent females. In analyzing these studies, the age of the child at
the time of treatment becomes an important factor.

Sanders: At the Seattle Marrow Transplant Group at Fred Hutchinson Cancer
Research Center, I have been following the patients that we have transplanted for both
aplastic anemia and acute leukemia between 5 and 10 years post-transplantation. The
numbers in that population are small. However, it is interesting in the aplastic women
who have been transplanted utilizing 200 mg/kg cytoxan as their regimen and 2 women
who also received procarbazine and ATG; we have previously reported 1 women who
had return of normal menses and a pregnancy following her cure for aplastic anemia.
She delivered a normal child. It appears in studying the whole group of women, of which
there are now 29 evaluable with follow-up times from 1 to 8½ years post-treatment for
aplastic anemia, that the 10 girls who were prepubertal at the time of their transplants did
develop normal ovarian function and went through menarche at a normal age, i.e. 12–14
years of age. I am gathering data on the men who were also transplanted during the same
period of time and who received the same high dose cyclophosphatide chemotherapy.
These men appeared to regain normal sperm counts somewhere between 2 and 5 years
following their marrow transplants. With respect to our leukemia patient transplants, it
appears as though one could say almost categorically that those patients prepared with
120 mg/kg of cytoxan and 1,000 rad total body irradiation are going to be sterile. However, there are a couple of exceptions. A girl who was 10 at the time of diagnosis of her
acute lymphoblastic leukemia and who was 13 at the time of transplantation became
pregnant 7 years post-transplant. She elected to have a therapeutic abortion at that time.
All other women that have been able to gather data on who were post-menarche at the
time of transplant appear to have gone through an early menopause. However, the follow-up time on these women is only 5 years, and there are 2 women that are between 5
and 8 years post-transplant that are on hormonal supplementation. The men appeared to
be azospermic with the exception of one who at 7 years post-transplant and who had
been followed serially for several previous years, had normal sperm counts, normal hormone levels, and fathered his own child. I think it's a matter of time.

Front. Radiat. Ther. Onc., vol. 16, pp. 156–166 (Karger, Basel 1982)

The Ethical Rights of the Child Patient

W.G. Bartholome

Department of Pediatrics, University of Texas Medical School at Houston,
Houston, Tex., USA

Introduction

I would like to begin my remarks with a warning. I am not a pediatric oncologist. In fact, unlike most of you, I spend very little of my time attempting the difficult task of responding to children with cancer. I am an outsider. The perspective I would bring to these remarks is a critical perspective. Some of you will find my remarks threatening and cynical.

Any discussion of the rights of children (particularly a discussion of the rights of children with life-threatening disease) is difficult to launch. For many adult members of our society, the concept of children's rights is suspect. From within the confines of a stable, intact family where living is shared and intimacy is the norm, heavy-handed concepts like legal or ethical rights seem strangely out of place. A professor of law once told me to think of legal rights as shields (to protect interests) or swords (to carve out that to which one is entitled). The idea that people who regularly make love and kiss and hug each other every morning and night might approach each other armed to the teeth in preparation for some adversarial conflict seems ludicrous. On the surface at least, it appears that to attempt to dissect and analyze spousal or parent-child relationships using the language or concept of rights is a little like using an axe where a butter knife might be appropriate.

Rights are the most powerful concepts in ethical dialogue or debate. They function much like trump cards in the game of bridge. Debates about obligation, duty or responsibility can end abruptly when a right is claimed. Historically, the language of human rights were the ideas that launched a revolution and served as the basis of the modern democratic state.

At this particular point in our social evolution, talk about ethics is virtually impossible without appeal to the concept of rights. The reasons for our attraction to rights talk are many, but the most basic explanation is that to many people, rights appear to be the only islands in a sea of ethical relativity. We live in a society in which basic questions like: 'What is a good life?' and 'What is the purpose or meaning of life?' are left to the individual to answer. We pride ourselves on our membership in a society in which all are free to live out their own life plan. Since few adult members of our society have any formal instruction or training in ethics, it is commonly assumed that this freedom demands that ethics be treated as 'relative'. In fact the principle of tolerance for the ethical beliefs of others is often proclaimed as a virtue.

Ethics is not relative. But it is difficult to achieve any kind of concensus about abstract and complex concepts like obligation, duty or responsibility. Since ethical rights are typically used to refer to distinct entitlements, and have a parallel development in law [6], they have become basic to any discussion of ethics. Although everything I will present could probably be expressed without reference to rights, I will fall into the trap of talking about rights primarily so that you might hear what is basically an argument about the ethical or moral 'standing' of children in our society, particularly those under treatment for life-threatening diseases.

Right to be Treated as a Person [3]

Those who would argue that the language of rights is clumsy, inappropriate and possibly dangerous when used to describe the intimate relating we call family are probably correct. However, I would argue that there is at least one respect in which the idea of a right seems required in description of parent-child relating. This basic right, once recognized within this relationship, becomes so much part and parcel of the day-to-day intercourse of family life that it is rarely visible – even to members of the family. Yet, when an infant or small child is taken out of the context of the family for example, when he/she is brought to a physician's office or a hospital; when a child is brought into contact with people, agencies or institutions outside the home – this basic right must constantly be recognized and respected.

The right to which I invite your attention is the right to be treated as a person – as a member of a community – as 'one of us'. The right can be stated in a variety of ways: the right to be treated as more than a pet or a possession; the right to be treated as more than the product or project of one's parents or society; the right to be treated as a radically unique, irreplaceable individual with interests and a destiny that are not those of one's parents or guardians.

This right can be appreciated by locking for the answer to the question: 'To whom do children belong?' [1]. Many adults are tempted to answer, initially, 'To their parents'. Some are uncomfortable with this response since it appears to reduce children to mere chattles. They flounder around for an answer: 'To the community', 'To the state', 'To the human race'. The problem many adults have in answering this question is symptomatic of the status problem of infants and children in our society. The obvious answer is that children do not 'belong' to anyone – unless one wants to argue that they belong to themselves or to a supreme being. If slavery is rejected on ethical grounds, there can be no 'belonging' or 'possessing' of human beings.

The Parent–Child Relationship and the Right to be Treated as a Person

Most parents can recall those experiences which precipitate – often ruthlessly and painfully – the realization that their children are radically separate persons. Classic descriptions of such experiences centered on seeing one's child off to school. However, often the precipitating event is an illness, a trip to the doctor, admission to a hospital, or – even more dramatically – a trip to an operating room. My oldest daughter was 4. Although she had left many hints of what was to come that hard day hit me like a ton of bricks. It was her hair. I had become accustomed to brushing it almost every night before she went to bed. I loved that hair and allowed myself to be caught up in its incredible beauty. That day as I walked in the door I remember being struck with how quiet it was. As I approached my wife I became aware of the fact that something was wrong, terribly wrong. We spoke with our eyes and as the tears welled up in her eyes and ran down her face, she handed me the envelope. My hands were shaking and I was aware of my heart pounding against my chest. It had a strange feel to it. It obviously contained something of considerable bulk, but it was strangely light. As I spilled the gold out into my hand, I stiffened as if it might burn me. I could not believe my eyes. I was stunned, paralyzed as if I had been shot. Slowly I became aware of the deep sadness that began to come over me like an icy fog. I held her hair in my hand and wept; big shaking sobs; out of control. I remember having felt that way only once before – in 1963 when I was told the President had been assassinated. Something deep inside me had broken, shattered; I felt as if I was about to unravel.

As I sat there, I became aware that Bridget was walking toward me. She was smiling. The self-administered hatchetjob she had performed on 'my' hair was barely noticeable. As she approached, she saw the pile of hair in my hands and the tears on my face. She immediately recognized that in cutting her hair she had broken me. We hugged. She comforted me with a reassuring pat and announced that Mom had called the beauty parlor to get a 'gooder' hair cut the next day. As we have grown up together we have talked about this episode occasionally. At age 12 she is now very much aware of the dramatic change in our relationship that occurred that day.

With my second daughter, the ruthlessness of my discovery of her as separate was almost unbearable. She was born 8 weeks early by emergency cesarian section and went not to her mother's arms nor to mine, but to an incubator in a neonatal intensive care unit. Her identity as a separate individual was painfully obvious when *her* doctor came to talk to me about *her* problems and *her* prospects. I remember watching her through that plastic. I have never been more aware of my impotence. I knew she was our newborn child, yet she was so much a stranger.

I tell these stories, I think, because I know of no better way to explain what I feel is so incredibly important about this most basic of rights: the right to be treated as a person.

The Right to be Treated as a Person and the Health Care Context

A full-blown philosophical defense of the right to be treated as a person is beyond the scope of our time here. Instead, I want you to examine some of the consequences of recognizing this right for health care professionals. If children have this right, then we must see and respond to them as persons, individuals like ourselves. When children are brought into the health care context they are not only torn out of the fabric of the shared living we call family, but rendered visible as individuals. New relationships are created. These relationships give rise to ethical obligations that can at times seem unbearable. The physician-child relationship, the nurse-child relationship, the psychologist – or social worker – or other professional-child relationship are created each with its own set of role-related duties; its obligations to an individual other; and its attendant responsibilities. Each member of what some have called the therapeutic community is then faced with the complex and demanding task of responding ethically to their new partner-in-relationship. Doing what is right by a child is a task that is frequently perplexing and occasionally overwhelming. What particular demands are placed on each member of the 'health care team' by this individual child who has just joined our hospital/clinic community?

Traditionally the enormity of this challenge has not been faced directly by the community of children's professionals. The demands have been seen as impossible. Many regard my argument as looking into a swamp of ambiguity, ignorance, and perplexity. Health care professionals are particularly intolerant of things like ambiguity and ignorance. The challenge of facing this impossible task of responding to children as persons is avoided. The tension is solved and the hurdle jumped by refusing to accept this burden. 'It is not for us to make these agonizing decisions. We are merely health care professionals. It is up to the parents. They bear the ultimate responsibility for their own children.' Often this claim is couched in the language of rights: parents have a 'right' to make these hard choices. Typically the concept of consent is borrowed from its appropriate framework in adult medicine and applied to these problematic situations. The concept of proxy consent has been accepted by the pediatric community, particularly the oncology community, with few (if any) reservations.

A Case in Point

I think it would be helpful to examine the argument of the oncology community in a specific case. In a recent article [4] *van Eys* presents an approach to a difficult case involving a 10-month-old infant with

leukemia. Before the infant's disease had been completely characterized and treatment begun, his parents elected to leave the cancer center
and take their infant to a faith healer. The author implies that such a
course of action is at least prima facie ethical since the parents 'chose to
substitute one mode of treatment with curative intent – chemotherapy –
for another – faith healing – thereby creating the dilemma'. He also
implies that in this case the dilemma is even more poignant since the
alternatives cannot be 'objectively evaluated'. If this case involved an
adult patient who declined chemotherapy to seek 'faith healing' most
of us would see no major ethical hurdle. We live in a society in which
adults are allowed to make such choices particularly if acting on such a
belief has no adverse affect on the interests of third-parties. *Van Eys*
claims: 'The fact that an infant is involved in this argument is not as
important as the argument itself.' I would claim that the fact that an
infant is involved must be seen as more important than the argument.
Why? If the infant in this case has the right to be treated as a person,
then the physician has a strict ethical duty to render to him competent
medical care. The physician also has ethical obligations to this particular infant (e.g., the obligation to 'do no harm') that derive from the
physician-patient relationship. The infant also has ethical claims
against the physician that are correlative of these duties and obligations. These duties, obligations and claims form the basis of the physicians responsibility to this infant. This responsibility does not disap-
pear because his parents have little or no faith in chemotherapy. The
physician in this kind of case will have great difficulty in ethically justi-
fying handing over the infant to a faith healer.

Van Eys rejects any claim to an 'absolute solution'. He states: 'No
doubt different physicians would have reacted and responded to this
challenge differently. The response is clearly dependent on the physician's own deep-seated spiritual beliefs'. He seems to be asking that
physicians be sensitive to the complexity of these hard cases. Physicians are asked to examine their 'deep-seated spiritual beliefs'. But,
there is a serious problem with this approach. The care to which an
infant is entitled should depend on neither the religious beliefs of his
parents nor on the 'deep-seated spiritual beliefs' of his professional
caretakers. A basic criteria of justice demands that our lives and our
welfare not be subject to the desires, opinions or spiritual beliefs of
others. *Van Eys* is right if he is making a claim about what does happen
in similar situations. An individual physician's response to this infant

may depend on his/her religious and/or ethical beliefs. However, that alleged fact about the way things are does not speak to the question of what ought to happen. I find it difficult to see any ethical justification for abdication of responsibility and leaving the infant's fate to be determined by his parents 'faith' and their alleged 'healers'. The only possible justification I can see for such a practice would be if the physician felt that the patient's prognosis with treatment was not significantly different from the prognosis with no treatment. In such a case, the responsibility of the physician to render care may be significantly diminished and the obligation to 'do no harm' may allow for the less harmful treatment approach proposed by the parents. But even this argument is highly questionable. Is not a dying infant entitled to more than the care that can be provided by a faith healer?

I find the spirit of the approach proposed by *van Eys* to be common among members of the pediatric oncology community. Members of this community seem very willing to allow parents a degree of power and authority over their children that is uncommon in other branches of the pediatric community. (Neonatology may well be a similar exception). Since I am an outsider, I can only speculate about why this happens. My speculations include characteristics of the community and their work.

First, I would speculate that at the present state of development, many members of the community see their approach to these patients as inherently ambiguous. In spite of impressive statistics, treatment continues to involve giving children agents which are often characterized as 'poisons'; performing radical surgical procedures; and exposing children to massive doses of ionizing radiation. In each individual case, the child is treated in this obviously harmful way in spite of considerable ambiguity about his/her future. It is difficult to find room for comfort when the prospect of providing benefit is so ambiguous and the treatment involves doing so much violence to the child. And each relapse makes it more difficult for the physician to claim that he/she is doing right by the child.

In fact, many members of this community are trained to take comfort in the fact that their work is directed not only at the individual child with malignant disease who may be their patient at any particular point in time, but directed at all children with cancer and to children of the future. Since it was established, the practice of pediatric oncology has been wedded to research. Thus, the oncologist can always seek, or at least intend, some benefit, some good. Not, perhaps, for this individual patient, but for others. The heavy burden of responsibility to each individual child is softened by conceptualizing one's task as having this broader purpose.

Secondly, I would speculate that a demand on the oncologist to shoulder the burden of ethical responsibility to each individual child – particularly in the past when most died in spite of treatment – would threaten to crush him/her. I have serious reservations, for example, about the ability of a physician to practice full-time thanantology. Perhaps, in an effort to create enough emotional space between themselves and the children, members of this community have also inadvertently created a moral space that protects them from the burden of ethical responsibility. I would think that this is particularly true of individuals who were attracted to the field not because of a burning desire to provide care to children with malignant disease, but to do research on cancer; to join in the 'war on cancer'.

Thirdly, I would speculate that the pediatric oncology community is just learning an important lesson about the practice of chronic versus acute care medicine. An acute sensitivity to the unique and idiosyncratic characteristics of an individual patient is rarely required in acute care medicine. In fact, much of the medical care that children need can be provided without explicit recognition of the individuality of each child. As care of the child with cancer has been transformed from care of dying children to the care of children with chronic disease, its practicioners will be forced to see and respond to their patients as individuals.

I think there is some evidence to support the claim that the pediatric oncology community is moving in the direction of recognizing a child's right to be treated as a person. One need only look at the behavior of those members of the community involved in the care of Chad Green. However, many practices persist which are highly problematic and which lend support to my criticism.

Few members of the pediatric oncology community have seen minor sibling-to-sibling bone marrow 'donation' as a serious ethical problem. From an ethical perspective using a sibling in this manner is highly ambiguous. Each individual case demands meticulous ethical justification. I suspect that acceptance of this highly questionable practice has become so widespread in part because members of this community have insulated themselves from the claims of individual child patients. Parental willingness to volunteer minor sibling bone marrow involves such an obvious conflict of interest that it should play almost no role in the justification of this practice. Yet, in many centers, parental permission is treated as a sufficient condition for the ethical justification of the practice. Other previously widely accepted practices include allowing parents to 'volunteer' their dying children for phase one studies. The standard argument was: 'It is their child. They are losing a child. It is for them to decide.' Again, the obvious conflict between the parents interests and those of the dying child seems to have been largely ignored. Another example is the practice of continually telling parents that they can decide to stop treatment at any time, particularly in the child who has experienced a relapse. Many parents find this practice confusing. The oncologist may be experiencing significant doubts about what he/she should do in such situations. But, telling parents it is for them to decide in order to avoid the responsibility and/or guilt involved is inappropriate. My final example is the common practice of asking parents to make the choice between two impossibly complex (for them) arms of a research protocol. Many parents are overwhelmed by such an approach and feel abondoned by the oncologist. Their ability to make such a decision is obviously suspect. One must also be suspect about the motivation of the oncologist who presents them with this obviously impossible task and then pats him/herself on the back for having worshipped at the altar of 'informed consent'.

I have argued that children, particularly children undergoing treatment for life-threatening illness, have a basic right which must be recognized and respected. I have called this the right to be treated as a person – an individual member of our community. I have argued that recognition of this right means that medical care decisions cannot depend solely on the individual tastes, preferences, desires or spiritual beliefs of their parents. I have also argued that its recognition involves a willingness to reject the concept of proxy consent or its more dangerous formulation: the alleged right of parents to make these difficult decisions.

When the life of a vulnerable, voiceless [5] (in the sense of being heard) member of our community is threatened by malignant disease, the most basic responsibility we have is to respond to him/her as an individual person. The child's parents do have the power to totally frustrate our efforts to respond to them. They have a degree of control over the child's life that no health care professional can have. Chad Green's parents defied a court order and took him to Mexico. Legal sanctions against them have been minimal. Chad Green is dead. But, the court's decision in Massachusetts was not some ludicrous exercise in futility. What Chad's parents did was illegal. It was also patently unethical. The court's decision is a clear and unambigious message to all in our society – a child with cancer ought not to be treated as the pet, or the possession, or the product or the project of his parents.

Summary

It is difficult, if not impossible, to adequately address the complex ethical dimensions of health care using the language of patients' rights. However, talk about rights has become such a popular way to express our ethical beliefs that it is important that we at least address questions like what are the ethical rights of cancer patients. A special problem arises when the patient involved is an infant or small child. Many adult members of our society are uncomfortable with the idea of children's rights. In fact, many analysts have argued that talk of such rights is nonsense. Within the context of the intimate, shared existence of the family, talk of children's rights may seem unnecessary or even inappropriate. The parent-child relationship has historically been defined ethically in terms of parental duties/obligations and children's needs. The author will argue that, regardless of how one resolves the debate about the rights of infants and children vis-a-vis their parents, it is essential in our present society that infants and children as patients in the health care context or in a variety of relationships outside the family be seen and responded to as right-bearing persons like ourselves. The author will argue that infants and small children in the health care context have the 'right to be treated as a person' and sketch some of the consequences of granting this right to children undergoing treatment for malignant disease.

References

1   Aiken; Lafollette (eds): Whose child: children's rights, parental authority and state power (Littlefield-Adams, 1980).
2   Bartholome, W.; Proxy consent in the medical context; the infant as person; in Research involving children (Appendix to the report and recommendations), The National Commission for the Protection of Human Subjects in Biomedical and Behavioral Research, DHEW publication No. 77–000573–26.
3   Bartholome, W.: The child-patient: do parents have the 'right to decide'? Proc. 8th Transdisciplinary Symp. on Philosophy and Medicine: The law-medicine relation: A philosophical critique. Philosophy and medicine series, vol. 10, (Reidel, Boston 1980).

4   Brody, B.; van Eys, J.: Faith healing for childhood leukemia, Hast. Cent. Report, *45:* 10–11 (1981).
5   Freedman, B.: On the rights of the voiceless. J. Med. and Phil. *3:* 196–225 (1978).
6   Houlgate, L.D.: The child and the state: a normative theory of juvenile rights (Johns Hopkins Press, Baltimore 1980).

W.G. Bartholome, MD, Department of Pediatrics, University of Texas Medical School, Houston, TX 77025 (USA)

Front. Radiat. Ther. Onc., vol. 16, pp. 167–176 (Karger, Basel 1982)

Impact of Cancer on the Family

John J. Spinetta

Department of Psychology San Diego State University, San Diego, Calif., USA

What exactly does the child with cancer experience from the point of diagnosis onward? How does he attempt to adjust to a life-threatening illness? Can the child's and family's attempts at mastery be measured, predicted, modified? Can the family's coping strategies be strengthened?

These are questions that are of major concern to both the medical and the psychosocial members of the health care team. As medical progress in recent years has increased the life spans of children with cancer, concern has shifted from what in the 1950s and 1960s had been a preparation for an inevitable death, to helping the child and family in the 1980s prepare for what is becoming an increased chance of *long-term survival*. With this increased survival rate, there has come a gradual change in research interests and concerns from focusing on issues relative to death, to focusing on life, with an increased interest in the *quality* of the child's life. What is called for, with this growing concern over the quality of the increased life span which medicine now provides a child with cancer, is a series of direct, highly objective, and systematic studies of the children in their attempts at selfmastery over an illness that has become less invariably fatal.

This paper will be an overview of the studies of our own research team. The purpose of the paper, while outlining some of the psychological repercussions of childhood cancer and some methods for resolving them, will be to underscore the fact that rigorous and well-controlled research is both possible and necessary in this area of increased concern.

Method

When our research team first began its efforts to study the child with cancer in 1969, an extensive literature had emerged devoted to helping both the professional and the parents to cope with what was then called a 'fatal illness' in the child. Helpful as these publications were, comments on the children themselves remained anecdotal and intuitive.

Our own concerns during the early 1970s centered upon learning, in a systematic way, from the children themselves the answer to one of the questions most frequently raised at that time regarding the child with a life-threatening illness: what does the child with cancer know about his or her illness and possible *death?*

We designed and conducted careful and rigorous studies of children with leukemia, aged 6–10 years. What we discovered was that the child in this age group appears to be very aware of the seriousness of the illness, even though the child may not yet be able to talk about the awareness in adult terms. Using projective measures to elicit stories from the children, we found that the leukemic children were significantly more preoccupied with threat to their body integrity and functioning than were the chronically ill children in the control group [7]. The leukemic children also expressed a greater degree of anxiety, both hospital-related and nonhospital-related, than did the controls. Using as a further projective measure a three-dimensional replica of a hospital room in an analysis of interpersonal distancing, we found that the children with leukemia in the study placed each of four figures in their hospital life (nurse, doctor, mother, father) at a distance significantly greater than did the matched control group of chronically ill children [8]. This distance increased even further with subsequent hospitalizations and nearness of death. It was inferred that the placement of the dolls by the dying children was reflective of a growing sense of psychological separation of the child from the hospital, both people and circumstances, for reasons specific to each child's reinforcement history.

In a very systematic and carefully measured manner, we were able to resolve what had become an accumulation of a set of contradictory attitudes about what the child actually knows about his illness and its possible fatality as the end draws near. Continuing in the same systematic research vein, we attempted to resolve the issue of whether awareness of their illness persists with the children with cancer when they are not in the hospital. We found that, like the leukemic children who are hospitalized, so too the leukemic children in remission, being treated as outpatients, were aware that theirs is no ordinary illness [5]. As progress was being made medically toward more effective treatment, the long-term survival rate was gradually increasing. By the mid-1970s, with the increased survival rate, there came a gradual change in focus from death to life, and an increased interest in the quality of life of the patient-child [2]. A new series of questions began to emerge relevant to the shift of focus of both medical and psychosocial concerns, from preparing for an inevitable death to helping the child and family prepare for what was becoming an increased chance of *long-term survival.*

Our group began systematic efforts to study *family communication patterns* relative to this changing focus. We conducted a pilot study of family and child communication patterns relative to the cancer, and found that the child's level of anxiety and distancing from meaningful figures in the illness environment was directly related to openness of family patterns of communication relative to the illness [6]. Those children whose mothers reported an *open and honest attitude within the family regarding the illness,* the treatments, and the potential effects of the illness, had a better self-concept, were less defensive, and placed family members *closer* in our projective three-dimensional measure than did those children whose mothers reported a relatively closed family attitude regarding discussion of the illness and its possible consequences.

It was the tenet of our current research group 4 years ago that the careful and rigorous study methods used earlier in the decade on issues and concerns relative to the child's awareness should be expanded to measure more precisely *other levels* of concern in the children with various types of cancer, levels based on increased chance for *long-term survival,* and which might prove to be quite different from what observation and anecdote had pointed to as the child's level of functioning.

Accordingly, we began a 4-year study. The twofold problem was to determine: first, how a child with cancer copes with a life-threatening illness; and second, how the child could best be helped to maximize *coping efforts* and obtain as full a quality of life as possible within the physical limitations imposed by the specific disease process itself.

One of the major features of the study was the testing of the children in their natural habitats: the home and the school. Prior rigorously designed studies had taken place in the hospital setting, and while such studies are important, they can give a skewed picture of the actual functioning of the child with cancer in normal day-to-day life events. Study method is detailed in *Spinetta* [3].

Results

Results of studies relative to objectives of the research project will be summarized at this point, in the following order: (1) pilot level interview of postdeath adjustment of prestudy families; (2) overall adjustment and adaptation of family members to the cancer; (3) school and the child with cancer; (4) development of 4 age-independent measures; (5) effects of disease variables on test responses; (6) survival and coping strategies and support mechanisms; (7) issues relevant to Mexican families, and (8) siblings of the child with cancer.

Effective Parental Coping following the Death of a Child from Cancer.

A semistructured interview schedule was administered to 23 sets of parents whose child had died of cancer, in order: first, to learn how well the parents had adjusted to life without their child; and second, to learn if a family's level of adjustment after the child dies could be related to variables occurring during the life of the child.

A *postdeath adaptation measure* was developed. Content analysis, based on judges' scores of the parents' current adaptational level, yielded a postdeath adaptation score. Conclusions were drawn regarding areas of strength and weakness in parental adaptation. But most critical to the goals of the study was sorting out variables which best summarized the parents' memories of their family during the life of the child, and demonstrating a significant relationship between these variables and the postdeath adaptation score. Those parents who were the most adjusted after the death of their child were (1) those who had a consistent philosophy of life during the course of the illness which helped the family accept the diagnosis and cope with its consequences, (2) those who had a viable and ongoing support person to whom they could turn for help during the course of the illness, usually the spouse, and (3) those who gave their child the information and emotional support the child needed during the course of the illness at a level consistent with the child's questions, age, and level of development [10].

The parents demonstrated to us that families can adjust to life without their child. Pathology and maladjustment are not inevitable. The parents also shared with us interview responses which allowed us to demonstrate the generally beneficial effects on the ultimate adjustment of the family members of such variables as a viable support system, open and responsive communication with the child during the course of the illness, and a commitment to one's basic life view. What we learned was that strengthening the family's own adaptive resources along the lines of the variables shown to be effective for postdeath adjustment might prove to be an effective intervention to be applied to the families prospectively.

Overall Adjustment and Adaptation of Family Members to the Cancer

At the end of the 3-year data collection portion of the study, an item-specific series of *criterion measures* was devised (the Family Adjustment Scale, or FAS), with objectively scoreable responses, in each of six categories: (1) whether the family unit meets the emotional needs of the *patient,* (2) whether the family unit meets the emotional needs of the *sibling(s),* (3) whether the family unit meets the emotional needs of the *mother,* (4) whether the family unit meets the emotional needs of the *father,* (5) whether the family unit meets the *medical needs* of the patient, and (6) whether the family unit meets the *day-to-day needs* of the family members. The item-specific criterion measure

(FAS) was given to the hospital-based extended health care team members to complete for each family which was taking part in the study. Results of the item-specific criterion measure responses (FAS) were correlated with earlier judgments of family and family member adjustment patterns. A significant correlation was found for each level of the 6 categories of concern between initial psychometrists' judgments and the health care team's responses to the FAS. Fathers fared less well than patients. Siblings fared least well of all.

School and the Child with Cancer

By far the most important and most far-reaching of the rigorously established findings from the study came from our efforts to study the children's responses to the cancer experience as exhibited in their attitudes and behaviors while attending school. While we found many signs of learning disabilities in the children with cancer when compared with the controls, a critical finding was the subtle but understandable reluctance of children with cancer to participate actively and fully in developmental challenges as they occur in their normal day-to-day school lives.

The school research program firmly and ably demonstrated that the children with cancer do *not* exhibit seriously maladaptive behaviors, and most certainly do *not* differ from their normal school-aged peers on the majority of attitudes and behaviors relative to school and to functioning while at school. They did exhibit specific learning difficulties, however, and they did exhibit a hesitation and reluctance to participate in tasks in a manner natural to children from the carefully matched control group. This reluctance and hesitation presents a major obstacle to the growth and development of the children with cancer into the fully active, confident, and competent participation in life's events which is critical if they are to become mature and competent adults [1].

Development of Four Age-Independent Measures

One of the difficulties encountered in attempting a study of children is the disparity in levels of development, with its accompanying lack of homogeneity in test responses. It is difficult to find a test which will apply as well to a child 6 years of age as it will to a child 18 years of age. One of the goals accomplished in the study was the development of four age-independent measures for use with children with cancer. As a measure of the child's, sibling's, and parent's overall level of adjustment, an age-independent set of criterion measures was developed, as noted above (FAS).

A second age-independent measure, developed specifically for the study of children's attitudes and behaviors relative to school and school functioning, is the Deasy-Spinetta Behavioral Questionnaire (DSBQ), also noted above.

A third age-independent measure, revised and applied specifically to the child cancer population, is the Kinetic Family Drawing-Revised (KFD-R), with an objective and easily exportable scoring procedure.

The fourth age-independent measure, applied from earlier work to our current population under study, is the Moral Scale for Children (MSC), a scale which applies the judgment of the children themselves, as well as the judgments of parents, teachers, and friends about the children, to the study of the child's level of morale and commitment to continued living exhibited despite the presence of cancer.

The value of instruments that are age-independent is that they allow comparisons of children at varying age levels and developmental maturity with one another, allow for children who grow into more mature levels to be compared with their own earlier responses, and allow for a more consistent judgment of child responses to the cancer experience with the purpose of intervening to help the children best strengthen their ability to deal with the cancer.

Effects of Disease Variables on Test Responses

One of the major variables of concern in the study was the effect on the child's functioning of disease stage, frequency of clinic visits, visibility of the illness, and level of pain or physical discomfort which the child was experiencing. Our research staff demonstrated in a detailed and specific manner the importance of disease stage, of visibility of effects of the treatment, of frequency of clinic visits, and of level of pain or physical discomfort felt by the patient, as variables affecting psychosocial adjustment and thus affecting responses to tests and instruments measuring that adjustment.

Survival and Coping Strategies, and Support Mechanisms

A further area of study and concern during the project was that of coping strategies and support mechanisms used by the children with cancer, their siblings, and their parents in their attempts at adjustment to and mastery of the cancer experience. A series of measures, both projective and objective, together with interviews of each family member, led to several conclusions regarding coping strategies and support mechanisms, prime among them the underlying strength in facing the task exhibited by the children as well as by the parents. The survival and coping strategies reported by parents in open-ended semistructured interviews were virtually identical to those reported by the parents whose children had died. The parents reported *spouse support* (or support of significant other, when spouse was missing), *religious belief* or basic belief in the fundamental meaning of life and life's events and occurrences, and *honesty with the children* in responding to their concerns about the illness, as their strongest and most viable sources for survival and mastery of the cancer experience.

With help, the children and the family members can achieve an effective quality of life within the physical limits set by the child's physical reactions to the specific disease process. Our studies are pinpointing support mechanisms which can lead to a more adaptive coping response on the part of the children, their siblings, and their parents.

Issues Relevant to Mexican Families

There are a number of children with cancer who live in Mexico, and are treated at our two local pediatric cancer treatment centers. It is of interest to us to determine if there are cultural differences in coping strategies and in the successful outcome of those attempts at mastery. We conducted interviews of the Mexican families to evolve working hypotheses for future studies of a longitudinal nature. What we found, in our pilot efforts, was that the families from Mexico, when compared to American families, have a tendency: to be less open with and understanding of the needs of the younger children relative to knowledge of the illness and its treatment effects, to rely less on spouses' mutual support and more on the support of friends and extended family, to have a much deeper and more abiding belief in the meaning of life and life events, which sustains them through the experience, and, because of this, to be more passive and pessimistic regarding efforts at treatment and cure of the child. These four working hypotheses will form the basis of future longitudinal efforts of our research team in determining needs of the Mexican families, so that we can best direct our efforts to helping the children adjust to and learn to master the illness and its treatment effects.

Siblings of the Child with Cancer

One final area of central concern to our research team has been and continues to be the response of siblings to the presence of cancer in a brother or sister. Very little has been written in the literature regarding sibling adjustment, and what has been written has been largely anecdotal and case study related. One of the major findings of our systematic study of siblings is how poorly the siblings fared when compared to their own brothers or sisters with cancer. The children with cancer fared worse than controls, and the siblings fared in some tests the same as the children with cancer, and in many tests worse. Not only did we find the siblings scoring at less adapted levels on some of the objective measures than their brother or sister with cancer, we also learned from the parents their concerns regarding the siblings. It is this combined set of findings, from the parents and from the siblings themselves, that prompts our *concern* over the children's continued growth and development, and our goal to minimize obstacles to that development.

What we have done with our study is call attention to the need, from a data base demonstrating that need. It is our hope that by making parents and health care professionals more aware of the very real needs of the siblings, we will be able to direct parental and professional efforts to helping the siblings with their attempts at adjustment [4].

Conclusions

If helping children, siblings, and parents adjust to the presence of cancer in the family is a goal, and if we are to succeed in helping family members toward that goal, then we must firmly believe that the *quality of life* is enhanced by maximal efforts devoted to living. While the presence of a life-threatening illness in a child may seem overwhelming and almost beyond understanding in its meaning or purpose, we have found that 'plugging away at life' in the face of this adversity becomes its own reward, both for the child and for members of the family.

Families suffer when a child is diagnosed with cancer. While each family is unique, some general findings from research efforts point to: (1) the need for an active and open level of communication about the illness, from the very beginning, with all family members, including the young children; (2) the need for continual updating of medical knowledge about the progress of the illness; (3) the need to maintain a healthy and positive attitude of hope toward the disease outcome and the treatment process throughout the course of the illness; (4) the need of family members to remain supportive of one another, and the need for hospital-based staff to extend the type of attentive concern and sharing of updated medical information which the family requires; (5) a greater attention by both parents and professionals to the needs of the siblings – the most neglected of the family members. Details regarding both our research and practical applications and intervention strategies are given in *Spinetta and Spinetta* [9].

In our research findings, the majority of children with cancer and their families are able to do well with proper help available at critical times of diagnosis and relapse, and at specific times of individual family needs throughout the disease course. These are not families exhibiting maladaptive behaviors; they are rather normal families undergoing a crisis, normal families whose underlying strengths and coping abilities can carry them through the course of the disease with a minimum of well-placed help.

It is the goal of our continued efforts to study how the children with cancer can be helped to maximize their coping efforts and obtain as full a quality of life as possible within the physical limits imposed by the disease process itself. It is our hope that by a *systematic examination* of how children cope, by a precise measurement of changing levels of awareness, concern, and effort on the part of the child, we can rise above the intuitive level in applying methods for the reduction of the emotional, social, and academic dysfunctioning in the child with cancer which may result from the illness and its treatment. It is our long-term hope that such systematic study, both by ourselves and by others, will prove successful in helping children with cancer to maintain a *normal quality* of life, continuing to participate as fully and successfully as they can in *family, community,* and *regular* school life.

References

1   Deasy-Spinetta, P.M.; Spinetta, J. J.: The child with cancer in school: teachers' appraisal. Am. J. pediat. Hemat./Oncol. *2:* 89–94 (1980).
2   Spinetta, J.J.: Adjustment in children with cancer. J. pediat. Psychol. *2:* 49–51 (1977).

3   Spinetta, J.J.: Adjustment and adaptation in children with cancer: a three-year
    study; in Spinetta, Deasy-Spinetta, Living with childhood cancer (Mosby, St. Louis
    1981.)
4   Spinetta, J.J.: The sibling of the child with cancer; in Spinetta, Deasy-Spinetta, Liv-
    ing with childhood cancer (Mosby, St. Louis 1981).
5   Spinetta, J.J.; Maloney, L.J.: Death anxiety in the out-patient leukemic child. Pedi-
    atrics 56: 1034–1037 (1975).
6   Spinetta, J.J.; Maloney, L.J.: The child with cancer: patterns of communication and
    denial. J. consult. clin. Psychol. 46: 1540–1541 (1978).
7   Spinetta, J.J.; Rigler, D.; Karon, M.: Anxiety in the dying child. Pediatrics 52:
    841–845 (1973).
8   Spinetta, J.J.; Rigler, D.; Karon, M.: Personal space as a measure of the dying
    child's sense of isolation. J. consult. clin. Psychol. 42: 751–756 (1974).
9   Spinetta, J.J.; Spinetta, P.D.: Living with childhood cancer (Mosby, St. Louis 1981).
10 Spinetta, J.J.; Swarner, J.A.; Sheposh, J.P.: Effective parental coping following the
    death of a child from cancer. J. pediat. Psychol. 6 (in press 1981).

J.J. Spinetta, PhD, Department of Psychology, San Diego State University,
San Diego, CA 92182 (USA)

Front. Radiat. Ther. Onc., vol. 16, pp. 177–183 (Karger, Basel 1982)

Nutrition of Children with Cancer

Jan van Eys

Department of Pediatrics, University of Texas System Cancer Center,
MD Anderson Hospital and Tumor Institute, Houston, Tex., USA

The questions around nutrition of the child with cancer have provoked answers propounded with much enthusiasm, conviction, and evangelical zeal. Unfortunately, in this cacaphonous dialogue, claims have been made for and against nutritional support for children with cancer that cannot be substantiated with data. In fact, many of the therapeutic claims were a priori unlikely. Confusion arose when ethical and scientific arguments were juxtaposed, and when support and primary therapy were confused. To feed a child is basic. The concept feeding is so basic that nurture and nutrition are derived from the same root [18]. To manipulate a basic need for secondary gains, however noble the motivation (such as cancer cure) creates deep-seated conflicts. This paper will attempt to place nutrition in perspective, and to indicate the facts actually available about nutritional support and cancer outcome. However, these facts will be summarized in the perspective of the process of cancer cure as is now proceeding in pediatric oncology.

Magnitude of the Problem

Malnutrition in childhood cancer is a serious problem because it is by no means rare. Furthermore, malnutrition is a frequently occurring complication at times of progressive incurable disease. Precisely because of the latter association, the post hoc, ergo propter hoc argument makes the (erroneous) feeling strong that if one could avert malnutrition, one could avert death.

Malnutrition in pediatric oncology occurs in two types. First there is the malnutrition associated with the diagnosis at presentation. Such malnutrition is generally acute in onset and is manifested primarily by anthropometric criteria. The primary and most important criterion is the weight for height, best expressed as percent of the 50th percentile for age and sex: $\leq$80% is evidence for severe malnutrition, while 81-<90% signifies marginal malnutrition. Because of the acute onset of cancer, most newly diagnosed children do not have hypoalbumin-emia [9, 16]. Later during the illness children often develop chronic malnutrition if therapy is ineffective. In such cases the marasmic or kwashiorkor picture is seen.

The incidence of initial malnutrition is significant. In a retrospective study among three institutions a weight/height ratio of $\leq$80% of the 50th percentile was seen in 3/42 and <90% in 10/42 children with lymphoma or histiocytosis; 6/88 at $\leq$80% and 20/88 at <90% for children with solid tumors; and 3/64 at $\leq$80% and 19/64 at <90% for children with leukemia [9]. All these children were newly diagnosed and not previously treated. In a prospective study at our institution 8% of all newly diagnosed children had overt malnutrition at first evaluation [11]. Among such patients, and among patients who have been treated with comparable therapy the incidence of malnutrition is not equal among all diagnoses. Especially Ewing's sarcoma and neuro-blastoma predispose to malnutrition [19, 20].

In recurrent disease the incidence of malnutrition is much higher and may approach 50% or more in children with predisposing diag-noses [20]. It was overall in excess of 40% in a group of children with tumors metastatic to and from bone [24]. Such malnutrition can be extreme. In neuroblastoma linear growth is often not impeded in spite of progressive disease and marked cachexia can result [17].

Consequences of Malnutrition in Childhood Cancer

The presence of malnutrition in childhood cancer patients by itself is not always accepted as a problem. In fact, the often quoted data that transplanted tumors progress slower in lean than in obese mice, or that carcinogens induce fewer tumors in lean than in obese animals [5] make many pediatric oncologists view the malnourished state as a po-tentially desirable one. However, two sets of observations argue against that view. First, though not most importantly, malnutrition appears to be a poor prognostic factor in overall outcome in children

Table I. Nutritional status at first referral for patients with solid tumors who achieved and maintained a complete remission, compared to patients who relapsed or did not achieve a complete response

Relapse status[1]	Nutritional status[2]				Statistical test and p value
	$\leqslant 80$	81–90	91–100	>100	
0	1	5	10	28	chi-square for trend
1	5	9	13	17	p = 0.01

[1] Codes for relapse status: 0 = achieved and maintained complete response; 1 = relapsed or did not achieve complete response.
[2] Expressed as percent of the 50th percentile.

newly diagnosed with cancer [9]. Table I summarizes illustrative data from that cooperative retrospective study. The extrapolation that vigorous nutritional intervention, therefore, will invariably improve the outcome is not valid, however. The ultimate outcome of the cancer depends on the effectiveness of the primary therapy and not on the vigor of the supportive therapy [22]. There are instances in which definitive therapy cannot be delivered because of the nutritional state of the patient, in such instances nutritional support will affect the outcome. However, in a randomized controlled prospective trial of intravenous hyperalimentation, such intervention did not change outcome in children who had cancer, metastatic to or from bone, though the infectious complications were related to the nutritional state [24].

A second consequence of malnutrition in the child with cancer is the same as it is in the child with any other disease. A malnourished child has inadequate growth, feels listless and poorly, is susceptible to infections when chronic malnutrition sets in, and may have delayed brain development when the malnutrition occurs at an early age. Were this to occur in any child, feeding should be an automatic response.

Causes of Malnutrition in Children with Cancer

The causes of malnutrition associated with cancer have been discussed frequently. *Costa and Donaldson* [7] generated a useful tabulation. *DeWys* [8] reviewed the malnutrition in the extreme state. Most causes are obvious: mechanical obstruction, nausea, vomiting, anorexia, postoperative ileus, malabsorption, and eventually the metabolic alterations from extreme starvation: cachexia. Two factors deserve a short discussion: the complications of chemotherapy and the psychological factors.

Current chemotherapy modes are becoming ever more vigorous. A recent review of newly diagnosed children at our institution who went into remission for at least 6 months showed marked weight loss among adolescents with osteosarcoma [11]. The common denominator was the severely debilitating chemotherapeutic regimen, with intraarterial cis-platinum as a major contributing factor. This drug is extremely nauseating. It was known from animal toxicity data to be predisposing to weight loss [10]. It can give severe renal toxicity [10, 13], with nutrient loss, resulting in hypomagnesemia [15]. Our own protocol clearly generates severe renal toxicity and even hypertension [12]. Therapy can be inordinately toxic and malnutrition-inducing.

Related to that phenomenon is the real and frequently overlooked problem of learned food aversion as a cause for anorexia and weight loss in children with cancer. *Bernstein* [1] demonstrated experimentally that learned food aversions in children receiving chemotherapy were rapidly induced. Using a rat-tumor model *Bernstein and Sigmundi* [3] could demonstrate that learned food aversion was a component in tumor anorexia, and that commonly used antitumor drugs could act as unconditioned stimuli to generate learned taste aversions in rats [4]. These data correlate well with the observation that children develop aversions to familiar and preferred foods in their usual diets when receiving gastrointestinal-toxic therapy [2] (table II).

Approaches to Malnutrition in Children with Cancer

Malnutrition, once established, can be treated independently of the presence of cancer or therapy [14, 22, 23]. A prospective study of nutritional management showed that maintenance of nutritional status is possible even during intensive therapy [14]. The simplest method that will be effective should be used. Intravenous hyperalimentation can be used and is safe and effective in children with cancer [20, 24], but indications must be clearly set [20]. Prevention is far more important. Con-

Table II. Aversions to foods in the diet [2]

	Number of patients showing aversions
Patients receiving GI toxic chemotherapy	16/33 (48%)
Patients receiving vincristine of no drug	3/25 (12%)

p <0.01.

tinued contact with a dietitian is vital [26]. The use of a kitchen on the hospital ward generates freedom to use a self-selected diet at self-selected times [17]. Learned food aversions must be avoided and recognized when they occur. Once psychogenic food refusal occurs, family therapy techniques may need to be used to reverse the complication [6].

Misunderstandings of the Problem of Nutrition and Cancer

Nutrition is basic to the care of any person, let alone a sick child. Having cancer constitutes no exception. The human does require a diet that contains a complexity of nutrients. Therefore, cells are vulnerable to metabolic disturbances from abnormal diet composition or from lack of dietary intake. That fact has been exploited in chemotherapy for a long time through the use of such agents as methotrexate, which is an antagonist to folic acid, and asparaginase, which starves tumor cells of the amino acid asparagine [21]. However, there is no magic diet that cures cancer. Nutritional therapy, in the sense of maintaining or restoring adequate nutritional status is a supportive therapy, and as such cannot create cures anymore than platelet infusions can effect cures in leukemia. In fact, were our primary therapy truly effective, supportive therapy need not be given [25].

Nutrition should be viewed for what it is: supplying the most basic need of children. No child has ever died from being appropriately fed, but many die of starvation. Oncology should not contribute to that statistic.

References

1 Bernstein, I.L.: Learned taste aversions in children receiving chemotherapy. Science *200:* 1302–1303 (1978).
2 Bernstein, I.L.; Bernstein, I.D.: Learned food aversions in cancer anorexia. Cancer Treatm. Rep. (in press).
3 Bernstein, I.L.; Sigmundi, R.A.: Tumor anorexia: A learned food aversion? Science *209:* 416–418 (1980).
4 Bernstein, I.L.; Vitiello, M.V.; Sigmundi, R.A.: Effect of tumor growth on taste-aversion learning produced by antitumor drugs in the rat. Physiol. psychol. *8:* 51–55 (1980).
5 Clayson, D.B.: Nutrition and experimental carcinogenesis: a review. Cancer Res. *35:* 3292–3300 (1975).
6 Copeland, D.R.; Friedrich, W.N.; Eys, J. van; Sullivan, M.P.: Psychogenic food refusal in pediatric cancer patients: diagnoses and treatment. Pediatrics. Am. J. Dis. Child. (submitted for publication).
7 Costa, G.; Donaldson, S.: The nutritional effects of cancer and its therapy. Nutr. Cancer *2:* 22–29 (1980).
8 DeWys, W.D.: Nutritional care of the cancer patient. J. Am. med. Ass. *244:* 374–376 (1980).
9 Donaldson, S.S.; Wesley, M.M.; DeWys, W.D.; Suskind, R.M.; Jaffe, N.; Eys, J. van: A prospective study of the nutritional status of pediatric cancer patients. Am. J. Dis. Child. (in press).
10 Guarino, A.M.; Miller, D.S.; Arnold, S.T.; Pritchard, J. B.; Davis, R.D.; Urbanek, M.A.; Miller, T.J.; Litterst, C.L.: Platinate toxicity: past, present, and prospects. Cancer Treatm. Rep. *63:* 1475–1483 (1979).
11 Jaffe, N.; Carter, P.; Carr, D.; Eys, J. van: Chemotherapy and nutrition in childhood cancer. Cancer Res. (in press).
12 Kletzel, M.; Jaffe, N.: Systematic hypertension: a complication of intra-arterial cis-diammine dichlorplatinum II infusion. Cancer *47:* 245–247 (1981).
13 Krakoff, I.H.: Nephrotoxicity of cis-dichlorodiammine platinum (II). Cancer Treatm. Rep. *63:* 1523–1525 (1979).
14 Rickard, K.A.; Kirksey, A.; Baehner, R.L.; Grosfield, J.L.; Provisor, A.; Weetman, R.M.; Boxer, L.A.; Ballentine, T.V.N.: Effectiveness of enteral and parenteral nutrition in the nutritional management of children with Wilms' tumor. Am. J. clin. Nutr. *33:* 2622–2629 (1980).
15 Schilsky, R.L.; Anderson, T.: Hypomagnesemia and renal magnesium wasting in patients receiving cis-platinum. Ann. intern. Med. *90:* 929–931 (1979).
16 Teitell, B.C.; Eys, J. van; Herson, J.: Comparison of technique of assessing malnutrition in children with cancer (Abstract 96). J. enteral parenteral Nutr. *3:* 514 (1979).
17 Eys, J. van: Nutritional therapy in children with malignancies: rationale, promises and problems. Cancer Res. *37:* 2457–2461 (1977).
18 Eys, J. van: Feeding the dying child: ethical decision in a new guise. Presented at: The child and death; Foundation of Thanatology Meeting, New York 1979 (to be published).

19 Eys, J. van: Malnutrition in children with cancer incidence and consequence. Cancer *43:* 2030–2035 (1979).
20 Eys, J. van: Nutritional management as adjuvant in pediatric cancer therapy; in Care of the child with cancer, pp. 86–92 (American Cancer Society, New York 1979).
21 Eys, J. van: Nutritional therapy in childhood malignancies – a historical perspective; in van Eys, Seelig, Nichols, Nutrition and cancer, pp. 91–110. (SP Medical and Scientific Books, New York 1979).
22 Eys, J. van: The effect of nutritional status on response to therapy. Cancer Res. (in press).
23 Eys, J. van: Cangir, A.; Carter, P.; Coody, D.: The effect of nutritional supportive therapy on children with advanced malignancy. Cancer Res. (in press).
24 Eys, J. van; Copeland, E.M.; Cangir, A.; Taylor, G.; Teitell-Cohen, B.; Carter, P.; Ortiz, C.: A randomized controlled clinical trial of hyperalimentation in children with metastatic malignancies. Med. Pediat. Oncol. *8:* 63–73 (1980).
25 Eys, J. van; Copeland, E.M.; Taylor, H.G.; Cangir, A.; Carter, P.; Cohen-Teitell, B.; Ortiz, C.O.: Supportive therapy with curative intent; in van Eys, Sullivan, The status of curability of childhood cancers, pp. 33–46 (Raven Press, New York 1980).
26 Wollard, J. (ed.): Nutritional management of the cancer patient (Raven Press, New York 1979).

J. van Eys, PhD, MD, Mosbacher Prof. of Pediatrics and Head, Department of Pediatrics, University of Texas System Cancer Center, MD Anderson Hospital and Tumor Institute, Houston, TX 77030 (USA)

Front. Radiat. Ther. Onc., vol. 16, pp. 184–189 (Karger, Basel 1982)

Unorthodox Methods of Treatment for Cancer

Helene G. Brown

Community Cancer Control, Los Angeles, Calif., USA

The 'freedom of choice' issue, the rights of patients to do with their bodies whatever they wish, the right to accept treatment or refuse it, the rights of parents to offer or withhold medical treatment for their children, the state's mandate to protect the health and welfare of all its citizens and the medical establishment using proven methods of treatment are locking horns. Societal problems are added to this equation. The cost of medical care is clearly too high. The lesser, cheaper diseases have been cured (infection, flu, pneumonia, TB, polio), leaving us with the more difficult and expensive diseases like cancer. Doctors have never lived in as chilly a climate, they are truly blamed for all these problems and at the same time expected to put scrambled eggs back in their shells. There is a 'my doctor is OK, but medicine overall stinks' mentality around us today. We are clearly inadequate in our treatment of cancer – surgery, radiation and chemotherapy. We know it is worthwhile because it works, but not always, and we too deplore the shortfall.

All of this is happening in the media, the marketplace, the courtroom, legislatures, clinics, hospitals, in California, in every state of the Union and internationally. The battle rages over the use of 'unorthodox, really "quack" methods of treatment': unproven, unconventional or alternative methods.

Quack remedies roughly fall into three categories: drugs, devices and diets.

Devices are by and large the same. The black box: it may be large or small, it may be black or birch, but it contains nothing but a complete circuit lighting the light and some dials and switches and is most prominently sold in rural areas of the country where access to clinics and medical centers is limited and difficult.

Drugs and diets in combination are the big money sellers today. Specifically Laetrile and the metabolic diet. More and more people are getting their health information from their friends and neighbors and from their local health food store rather than through physicians. Let me demonstrate what is happening by relating a recent experience, but first my disclaimer – I am not against health food stores, or healthy foods. I part company with the health food store operators when they diagnose illness and tell me what to do for it. I am not against Laetrile or the metabolic diet if they work. I am against anything wherein a claim is made that is brazenly false and no evidence is offered to indicate otherwise. I think this is enormously wrong and is a new dimension in murder. In cancer, truly, fakes can be fatal. Knowing that I would be speaking with you today, I went into my neighborhood health food store, picked an assortment of books from the shelf, placed them on the counter and asked if there was anything here that could help my problem. It was obvious what my problem was. One book was 'Does Dr. Max Gerson have a true cure for cancer?' Dr. *Gerson* was a practicing physician in New York City. You may recall a book written by *John Gunther* called 'Death be not proud', in which he describes his son's fight against a terminal brain malignancy. There is a chapter in the book that describes his sons's time under the care of Dr. *Gerson*. Surely the place for the child then was at home eating all the whipped cream and ice cream and Milky Ways that one could find, being offered the caring and comfort of his family, making dying better – instead of suffering the indignities of a carrot juice diet that offered only false hopes. Another book talks about the 'grape cure' for cancer and is essentially the same. One fasts for 72 h and then commences a diet of grapes until the cure is complete: grape juice, grape pits and grape husks, but no fermented grapes. The best seller of them all discusses 'live vegetable juices'. On page 132 you can find, in alphabetical order, any ailment that you might have and the formula for the care of that ailment.

The operator of the store said, 'yes, there is something that will help you in these books...and before you go to a doctor...' – please understand, she knows that I have cancer and is suggesting that *before* I go to a doctor – 'who will cut, burn and poison you' (that is the vernacular for surgery, radiation and chemotherapy) 'you should try Laetrile and the metabolic diet that goes along with it.' I asked her if she sold Laetrile and she said, 'it is illegal to do so, but I have some tablets and some apricot seeds that will give you amygdalin' (the active ingredient in Laetrile). She offered me 100- and 500-mg tablets and a bag of apricot seeds. I asked about purity, about the manufacturer's name and she assured me that I was buying the best, even in the absence of labels. I asked about dosage and she said: 'take as many as you can tolerate'. When I asked her to describe what she meant, she described the symptoms for cyanide poisoning, which indeed occurs when Laetrile is ingested orally. Many patients enter emergency rooms having these symptoms due to overdose of Laetrile. Then she commenced to review with me the necessary metabolic diet that accompanies Laetrile therapy.

This is the very same information that took the lives of both Chad Green and Steve McQueen. Chad Green, you will recall, was 20 months old at the time of diagnosis of acute lymphocytic leukemia (ALL). Chemotherapy treatments were started and remission achieved. The therapy conflicted with the parent's choice of treatment and so they took him off chemotherapy. When they refused to resume chemotherapy, the treating physician petitioned the courts for appointment of a temporary guardian to consent to treatment. In the transcript of the court, the following statement is made: 'Although Chad Green would have had an 80% chance of total cure if chemotherapy and never stopped, cessation of chemotherapy reduced his chance of cure. Laetrile had caused chronic cyanide poisoning and megadoses of vitamin A had caused hypervitaminosis A' [1]. After numerous court appearances, the parents left the country with their son, put him in the hands of Dr. *Ernesto Contreras* in Mexico, and Chad Green succumbed. The court made four statements of fact and conclusions: (1) in spite of the public attention that Laetrile has generated, there is virtually no evidence supporting its efficacy as an anticancer drug, either alone or in combination with other substances; (2) that Laetrile therapy is dangerous in that the quality of Laetrile available in the United States is extremely uneven and generally terrible; (3) that Laetrile can cause acute or chronic cynide poisoning. Accumulations of hydrogen cyanide can cause progressive damage to the brain and the nervous system and can lead to deafness, blindness and gait problems, and (4) that the principal components of metabolic therapy are themselves toxic in the dosages prescribed, and determined that every component of metabolic therapy had already harmed or could potentially harm Chad Green.

While Steve McQueen's diagnosis of mesothelioma was not as hopeful as the ALL of Chad Green, he undoubtedly died a worse death than necessary. The metabolic diet that he adopted was 180 degrees from being beneficial to a cancer patient and indeed was actually harmful. The diet calls for the following:

(1) No meat, fish or fowl. These are the major sources of absorbable iron in the American diet. Their lack results in a high frequency of iron deficiency and iron deficiency anemia, *thereby harming cancer patients*.

(2) No dairy products. These are the main sources of calcium in the American diet. Lack of adequate calcium damages bone maintenance, *thereby harming cancer patients*.

(3) No animal protein. Animal protein is the exclusive source of vitamin B_{12} in the American diet, with the exception of B_{12}-fortified foods and microorganisms such as seaweed. Lack of this vitamin interferes with basic biochemical processes in normal tissue, *thereby harming cancer patients*.

(4) Increased ingestions of fruits and vegetables. Such a diet is high in bulk and low in calories, just opposite to the needs of cancer patients. In addition, it is low in needed animal protein, thereby *harming cancer patients*. Furthermore, fruits and vegetables contain varying quantities of the enzyme B-glucosidase which releases cynide from Laetrile, thereby making cyanide poisoning almost certain. Thus, the nutritional and metabolic program of Laetrile proponents is perhaps as unhealthy for cancer patients from the nutrition and metabolism standpoint as it is possible for the mind of man to conceive [2].

Let us take a look at some of the major concerns that we must have. Laetrile is neither safe nor effective. It cannot be approved by the FDA for use in human cancer. In the light of this fact, is there a valid claim for 'freedom of choice'? Clearly, the answer is 'no'. We have a limited freedom of choice in our country. You may choose how to dress, what school to go to, what church to support, what meals to eat, etc. But the moment a law is passed, we have forfeited our freedom of choice. We cannot choose to run a red light. We cannot choose to tear our house down and build a gas station. The zoning laws interfere with our freedom of choice. We cannot buy a fraudulent share of stock on the NYSE. The SEC governs that for the protection of the people. Likewise, we cannot buy a drug that is neither safe nor effective. The 'freedom of choice' argument falls of its own weight. Is there a valid claim that the 'medical trust' in the United States does not allow a cancer cure like Laetrile to be marketed, for they will lose their lucrative livelihood? I cannot accept that as there is no historical precedent for such a claim. Figured in today's dollars, the 'medical trust' should not have allowed a vaccine for polio to be marketed or the INS and streptomycin that cures TB. These would be far more lucrative diseases to have around than cancer. This did not happen with these and countless other examples, so one cannot accept that claim today in the field of cancer.

Scientific decisions are today being made in courtrooms and in legislatures. When a judge or legislator declares that a drug be legally approved for sale over the objections of scientists and the FDA, it becomes enormously wrong and should not be allowed to continue.

Quackery is simply a question of who do you believe?

The health team must understand and accept that cancer patients are fearful of death or of physical or mental incapacity. They need to believe, especially when their condition is deteriorating, that they will not be abandoned by medicine, that the health team is credible, that it knows what it is doing and that it is doing all that can be done. They must know that though cancer may not always be curable, it is always treatable. This takes *time* and the offer of time and support must be real: time to explain all the patient wants to know, to explain the next steps, to explain to the family, to discuss expectations, to establish credance and belief in what the doctor and his team have to offer, to explain that Quacks are rampant, to indicate competence and understanding, and to show interest. Use the team, the nurse, the social worker, the psychologist, the hypnotist, the health educator, whatever the patient and his family need in a people-to-people show that never leaves the patient feeling abandoned. Time to touch, show interest, feeling and support.

Stand up and be counted when a Laetrile legislation bill is introduced on the floor of your legislature and force the enactment of stringent laws to combat this treachery. It is clearly our responsibility, yours and mine, to offer the patient and his family all possible means of support.

When *Edmond Burke* said the following, it was as true as it is today: 'The only thing necessary for the triumph of evil is for good men to do nothing.'

References

1   Norris, J.A.: Am. J. Law Med. *6:* 151–171 (1980).
2   Herbert, V.: Letter to the editor J. Am. med. Ass. *240:* 1139 (1978).

H.G. Brown, MD, Executive Vice President, Community Cancer Control,
5800 Wilshire Blvd, Los Angeles, CA 90036 (USA)

Front. Radiat. Ther. Onc., vol. 16, pp. 190–191 (Karger, Basel 1982)

Discussion

Audience: Dr. *Wilbur,* can parents look at the hospital records of drugs administered, blood pressure, and so on?

Wilbur: We have an open chart system in our unit and encourage patients and their family members to read the chart, look at laboratory results, look at medications being given and become knowledgeable about everything that is being done, to ask questions and for us to ask them questions.

Audience: Do many hospitals follow this procedure?

Wilbur: Some hospitals do. I think the tradition from years ago has been to not allow ready access to the medical records. That is slowly changing.

Bakey: Dr. *Barholome* mentioned the idea of the child giving consent for care, treatment, procedures, etc. Are any of you familiar with any hospital setting that is developing informed consent forms or procedures for children, and what ages are you looking at for that being a reasonable plan?

Bartholome: I do not believe that we ought to put children in an unenviable situation of trying to consent to their own medical care. You are in a kind of double jeopardy when you are a child. I do think that it is very important to look at the notion of consent in this area. I do not think that the concept has any role at all in situations where the patient is a child. I think that we have to replace that concept with other concepts, and that is clearly starting now in the area of research. The National Commission for Protection of Human Subjects recommended to the Secretary of Health, Education and Welfare, and it was adopted by the Secretary that it be recognized that a parent cannot consent to the involvement of his or her child in research – that a parent may give permission for such involvement but that must be a way of distinguishing permission from consent. In certain situations, even though the child does not want something to be done, it may be necessary to use power and violence and do it to the child. That happens all the time. I am not saying that that is absolutely wrong. I am saying that it is wrong insofar as it is doing violence to a child, and you better have a very good reason for doing it. I am not at all sure that research is enough of a reason to do it. We ought to look at that question. I think that you start involving children in real-life decision making, maybe not in a controlling way, probably as early as ages 5–7. What they say between then and the time they are 18 should be listened to. It may not be the controlling thing that makes the decision, but as the child gets older decision making should clearly be more and more vested in the child. Some people would argue, and I would support the notion, that a child of 12 may very well be ready to make important decisions. We certainly would now allow a child of 12 to make decisions in a vacuum. But if a child of 12 understands what is going on, has been informed, and his reality includes the decision that you are talking about, and he makes the decision to say no, it is difficult to overrule that. The problem is that one has to distinguish between the legal concepts of consent and ethical concepts of consent. The legal concept is a very heavy-handed absolute-limit kind of thing. The ethical concept can be much more flexible and fluid.

Oppenheimer: I am a retired pharmacist and have a question for *Helen Brown.* There is a law that legalizes Laetrile in the state of California. Fortunately, many restrictions have been placed upon its use. Registered oncologists are the only ones who legally can prescribe it, and it can only be dispensed through very special methods and places. On the 25th of this month (March, 1981) there may be discussion and passage on a lifting of the restrictions. Are you familiar with this?

Brown: Yes, the bills legalizing the manufacture, sale and use of Laetrile have now been passed in 22 states in the union. In 21 of those states they have not had very much success with it or they will not have because it is still forbidden from interstate commerce, and in some states they simply do not grow enough apricots to make the product. In California we have a different situation. Last year the bill came into the legislature to freely allow Laetrile to be sold, marketed and used in the state of California through health food stores, practitioners and others. We were able to tighten up that bill before it was passed. We have a real problem. Because of the governor's support for that bill, it was passed. In order that the bill be watered down there were some of us who fought very hard to have the privilege of using Laetrile reserved to board-certified oncologists. We knew at that time that Senator *William Campbell* from Whittier would be back again this year with a bill to loosen up that which has already been passed. I am glad, Dr. *Oppenheimer,* that you brought it to all of our attention. Certainly, a loosened-up Laetrile bill will, indeed, be on the floor of the legislature this year, and again I urge all of you when you hear about it or read about it to approach your legislators. Unfortunately, laws good tools, and we really can live without a law that so brazenly reduces a scientific judgement to the trading back and forth of the legislators in California.

Audience: I think that it would be wonderful if all pediatric centers could have the type of setting that you, Dr. *Wilbur* and Ms. *Bivalec* have brought out because I do not know whether everyone here realizes that this is protective of our immune defenses by relieving stress and making it better for the patient and the family, they are better able to respond to the therapy that is given to them.

Sakai: How long has the pediatric oncology ward been around?

Wilbur: The original unit was developed at Children's Hospital in Boston in the late 1940s. Since that time there have been a number of units established all over the country, the one at M.D. Anderson being one of the early ones.